NATURAL
FOOT
CARE

HERBAL TREATMENTS, MASSAGE, AND EXERCISES FOR HEALTHY FEET

STEPHANIE TOURLES

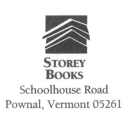

STOREY BOOKS
Schoolhouse Road
Pownal, Vermont 05261

DEDICATION

To my parents, Mike and Brenda Anchors,
for their guidance and patience, and for instilling in me the
courage to pursue my lifelong dreams.

*The mission of Storey Communications is to serve
our customers by publishing practical information that encourages
personal independence in harmony with the environment.*

Edited by Pamela Lappies and Julia Rubel
Text design and production by Sue Bernier and Erin Lincourt
   (based on original design by Carol Jessop, Black Trout Design)
Production assistance by Jennifer Jepson
Cover design by Carol Jessop, Black Trout Design
Cover art by Laura Tedeschi
Illustrations by Kathy Bray and Laura Tedeschi
Indexed by Hagerty & Halloway

Printed in the United States by R.R. Donnelley
10 9 8 7 6 5 4 3 2 1

Library of Congress Cataloging-in-Publication Data

Tourles, Stephanie L., 1962–
    Natural foot care / Stephanie Tourles.
        p.   cm.
    "A Storey Book."
    Includes bibliographical references (p.).
    ISBN 1-58017-054-4 (pbk.)
    1. Foot—Care and hygiene—Popular works. 2. Foot—Wounds and injuries—Treatment—Popular works. 3. Foot—Massage—Popular works. I. Title.
    RD563.T68   1998
    617.5'85—dc21   98–19917
                                                                CIP

CONTENTS

ACKNOWLEDGMENTS

I'd like to extend my gratitude to the following people who shared their talents and expertise to help bring this book to fruition: My husband, Bill, for his loving support and encouragement when writing this manuscript seemed a daunting task and for enduring scores of take-out dinners; my grandparents, Earl and Phenie Ashe, for passing on their wisdom about the world of growing things and for giving me an incredibly green thumb; my grandmother, Grace Anchors, for her help in obtaining information on Cherokee Indian herbal healing methods; my mother-in-law, Nancy Sullivan, for her love of the green world and her inspiration to create all things beautiful; my editor, Pamela Lappies, for her book idea and for asking me to give it life; Andrea Murray, for her interesting twist of combining reflexology with herbalism; William Rossi, D.P.M., for his refreshing and insightful views of the human foot and its care; Carol Frey, M.D., for her article and research materials; Walter Pedowitz, M.D., Board Member of the American Orthopaedic Foot and Ankle Society, for his expertise and humor; Sherry Ketchum of Birkenstock; LeeAnne Sullivan, owner of Cosmetique in Hyannis, Massachusetts, for the fabulous pedicure and entertaining foot care stories; Ruthann Foss, for her generous nail care information; Jean Argus, for her recipe and herbal supplies; Julie Bailey, for her calendula oil recipe; Lisa Hanley, for information on my favorite Dr. Scholl's Exercise Sandals; David Teufel of L.L. Bean, for information on Bavarian Wool Clogs; David Meyer, for Clarence Meyer's herbal folklore recipes; Rebecca Slama, for Easy Spirit shoe information; Carole Imperiale of Schering-Plough HealthCare Products, Inc., for foot care brochures; The American Orthopaedic Foot and Ankle Society, for their research materials and for answering my many questions; The American Podiatric Medical Association, for foot care information; and the Pedorthic Footwear Association. Lastly, thanks, Douglas, for the joy, the laughter, and the hope.

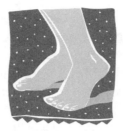

INTRODUCTION

THE HUMBLE FOOT

To be honest, when my editor, Pamela Lappies, called me to ask whether I'd be interested in writing a book on natural foot care, I was both pleased and disappointed. Although I was excited that my publisher wanted me to write another book the first words out of my mouth were, "An entire book dedicated to feet? Who wants to read about feet?" In my first book, *The Herbal Body Book* (Storey Publishing, 1994), I wrote one chapter about natural foot care and I thought that was plenty. But, as I started to ponder the topic in more detail and began talking to everyone I came in contact with about the subject, I soon realized that caring for the feet is a sorely neglected part of everyday personal hygiene — leading, of course, to problems resulting from sore, neglected feet.

Anywhere you look or listen, be it magazines, television, radio, retail stores, or mail-order catalogues, you're bombarded with beauty industry media revolving around hair, skin, and nail care; diet and exercise programs; thinner thigh and anticellulite creams; hair color to restore your lost youth; or promises of whiter and brighter teeth in seven days. The humble foot is an often ignored body part. Products for the feet make up a very small percentage of sales in the health and beauty segment of the market. Why?

I have an inkling that one reason is because the foot is one of the least–seen parts of the body. It's not glamourous, it rarely gets shown off, so it doesn't receive the attention that other body parts do: The foot doesn't get styled, brushed, or buffed, and it doesn't need whitening or slimming. It's not used for attracting a mate (unless, that is, your mate of choice has a foot fetish). The foot is usually not exposed to the public, except during the summer months, when many people would rather hide their feet than showcase them. I've never even heard of a contest for the most beautiful feet, have you? I bet even beauty queens don't have beautiful feet — especially after forcing them into uncomfortable, 3-inch heels for hours, perhaps days, on end.

The average person's foot is just plain unattractive and taken for granted. Maybe you occasionally use a pumice stone to grind down your calluses, cut your toenails, massage lotion into your heels, or possibly even paint your nails. But the majority of the time you ignore your feet and simply stuff them, day after day, into ill-fitting shoes and expect them to feel just peachy!

There's actually very little literature about foot care available to the public, unless you know where to look or have an interest. But I hope to change that with this book. In it you will find topics on everything from nutrition for healthy feet to medical problems and their solutions, to advice on proper footwear, professional and home pedicures, and massage. I hope it will be an eye-opening book for you and make you think twice about your "dogs" and begin to appreciate them. Foot care shouldn't be a chore. With all the recipes in this book, you'll soon look forward to "feet treats" as a way of unwinding or of perking up.

I should mention that while I was doing research on the herbal foot care recipes presented here, I made and experimented with so many salves, lotions, creams, and scrubs that by the end of my creative period, I took notice of the condition of my skin and nails. Everything was positvely glowing — particularly my feet, which had been the focus of all that pampering. I had incredibly silky smooth skin everywhere; even my normally callused feet were soft. Getting into a daily habit of slathering yourself with beneficial, handmade herbal products really pays off!

I hope the recipes in this book appeal to you. Try as many recipes as you can. You'll have fun, learn a lot, and your feet will thank you.

Blessings of health to you and yours,

Stephanie L. Tourles

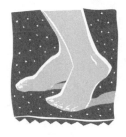

CHAPTER 1

FOOD FOR THE FEET: BASIC NUTRITION FOR HEALTHY FEET AND TOENAILS

"Food for the feet": Does that mean there's a special diet that can transform ugly duckling feet into beautiful swans? No, not completely, I'm sorry to say. However, I do know that a whole foods, natural diet contributes greatly to overall health, cultivating glowing skin and healthy feet and toenails. Combine this diet with proper footwear, exercise, plenty of water, and exposure to fresh air and safe amounts of sunlight, and you're on your way to truly fabulous feet.

Just what types of foods constitute a whole foods diet? Normal, everyday foods do, actually. But, it's just these types of foods that we have let slip from our diet and gradually replaced with refined, overprocessed, preservative laden, sugary food substitutes. If we ate whole, unprocessed food, the way many of our great–grandparents did, we'd probably be a lot healthier. They ate foods the way Mother Nature served them up: fresh, unprocessed, and in season from the wild and from nearby gardens or farms. Now, I'm not advocating that everybody dig up their lawns and start farming (though we'd all probably be a lot healthier if we did). It is possible to eat a natural diet by going to the local grocery store. It just means spending more time in the produce section, skipping the junk food aisles, and purchasing lean meats, whole grains, and low-fat dairy products. This chapter gives a quick overview of basic foods and healthful eating, along with a few of my favorite recipes for vitamin and mineral supplements.

A WHOLE FOODS DIET: CARBOHYDRATES, PROTEINS, AND FATS

The three basic food categories, carbohydrates, proteins, and fats, are commonly called macronutrients. They are so named because they comprise the greatest portion of the human diet. Macronutrients provide calories for fuel and help to regulate body heat.

Carbohydrates

This is probably my favorite food category. I love to eat freshly baked bread, fruit salad, popcorn, wild rice, and butternut squash. Carbohydrates are found in foods rich in starch and natural sugars. They're chock-full of vitamins and minerals and supply power to your brain and muscles. They are to your body what jet fuel is to a rocket — pure energy!

Carbohydrates come in two forms: simple and complex. Simple carbohydrates are plentiful in foods such as honey, molasses, maple syrup, table sugar, and highly refined foods including cake, candy, and cookies. These foods are broken down quickly by the body and can produce a "rush" of energy but should only be eaten sparingly as they are nearly pure simple sugar. Fresh and dried fruits are far superior in nutritional quality and are a recommended part of a healthy diet, albeit they are also loaded with simple sugars.

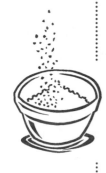

Just remember: if it's sweet, it's packed with simple carbohydrates. The exception to this rule is milk, which is not all that sweet but has plenty of simple sugars in the form of lactose.

Complex carbohydrates should be the mainstay of your diet. According to the United States Department of Agriculture (USDA), 55 to 60 percent of daily calories should come from complex carbohydrates. They provide loads of vitamins A, B complex, and C, which are crucial to healthy skin and circulation. These vitamins are found primarily in whole grains, beans, and vegetables such as squash, carrots, onions, corn, and potatoes. (Green vegetables are comparatively low in carbohydrates but are high in vitamins, minerals, and fiber.) Complex carbohydrates provide another bonus: plenty of fiber, necessary for a healthy digestive system. Another benefit is that they're generally low in calories as long as you stay away from fatty toppings like butter and sour cream.

The USDA Food Guide Pyramid recommends 6 to 11 daily servings of grains, rice, and pasta, 3 to 5 servings of vegetables, and 2 to 4 servings of fruits. Those are easy and delicious goals to reach every day!

Proteins

The fish you had for dinner last night or the tofu in the stir-fry you ate for lunch today consists primarily of protein. Protein is found in every cell of your body and is vital to healthy hair, skin, and feet. It is broken down by the body into components called amino acids, which are used to form muscle, repair damaged tissue, grow new hair and nails, form enzymes and hormones for various functions, and produce antibodies to combat disease and increase metabolism.

RECOMMENDED COMPLEX CARBOHYDRATES

Beans, peas, lentils, peanuts (these also contain significant protein)
Whole grain rice
Whole grain bread/pasta
Whole grain cereals (barley, oatmeal, buckwheat groats, amaranth, quinoa, yellow grits, millet, etc.)
Chestnuts
Sprouted seeds (clover, wheat, sunflower, alfalfa, soybeans, etc.)
Barley grass, wheatgrass
Blue-green algae (spirulina) and green algae (chlorella) — also high in vegetable protein
All fruits — fresh and dried (fruits contain simple and complex sugars)
Vegetables (such as carrots, onions, squashes, corn, potatoes, cabbage)

Your diet should consist of approximately 20 to 30 percent protein, depending on your level of activity and health condition. The greater amount is primarily required by body builders, elite athletes, pregnant and lactating women, surgical patients, and those with physically demanding jobs (tree climbers, workers involved in heavy construction, or stone masons, for example).

A protein deficiency is rare in the United States, but a lack of sufficient protein in your diet can result in opaque white bands appearing across the fingernails and toenails and cause them to become thin, dry, or brittle.

The USDA Food Guide Pyramid recommends 2 to 3 servings per day of meat, poultry, fish, beans, eggs, or nuts and 2 to 3 daily servings of milk, yogurt, or cheese. These two groups provide your body with vitamins A and B complex, iron, zinc, copper, and calcium.

RECOMMENDED PROTEIN SOURCES

Beans, peas, lentils, peanuts
  (these also contain signifi-
  cant carbohydrates)
Tofu
Texturized soy protein
Soybeans
Tempeh
Soy milk
Soy burgers
Nutritional yeast
Eggs
Lean dairy (milk, yogurt, cheese)
Nuts, including almonds, brazil
  nuts, hazelnuts, and walnuts

Seeds, such as sesame, pump-
  kin, or sunflower
Blue-green algae (spirulina) and
  green algae (chlorella) (also
  high in carbohydrates)
Seafood
Lean poultry
Lean beef
Lean pork
"Wild" meats, such as venison,
  buffalo, antelope, duck,
  squab, or rabbit

There are plenty of alternative protein sources to choose from today if you are a vegetarian or merely wish to vary your diet. I happen to prefer vegetable protein over animal protein, never have been a big fan of meat, and regularly include grilled soy burgers and fruity soy smoothies as part of my diet. Since I live by the ocean, I do enjoy a piece of fresh fish about once a week.

Fats

Good fats, bad fats, monounsaturated fats, polyunsaturated fats, saturated fats, essential fatty acids, omega-3 fatty acids — this fat business can get a bit confusing. Any way you look at it, the dietary nutrient fat has a bad reputation. It's undeserved: Fat is a necessary part of a healthful diet, as are carbohydrates and proteins. It serves to insulate your organs, support and contour your skin, and facilitate digestion and absorption of the fat-soluble vitamins A, D, E, and K. It makes your skin pliable and gives you a dewy glow. Only when eaten in excess does it become a problem. Too much of any good thing can be detrimental, even extra-virgin olive oil!

Excess fat in the diet is one of the leading causes of obesity and coronary heart disease in this country. Being overweight can lead to foot problems such as fallen arches, bunions, excess perspiration and odor, bone misalignment, and weakened feet in general. The added weight delivers more shock per step to feet, resulting in more wear and tear than the average pair of "dogs" were made to withstand.

The average American gets about 35 to 40 percent of daily calories from fat, though the USDA recommended amount is approximately 15 to 25 percent, depending on activity level and health condition. Is it any wonder we have such a high obesity rate in this country?

Fat by itself doesn't have much flavor. However, when fat is added to other food the result is a rich, smooth mouth feel and full-bodied taste that is both delicious and addicting. While a little fresh butter every once in a while is part of a healthful diet, problems arise when you put butter in and on everything from bread to veggies to cream sauces.

The USDA Food Guide Pyramid recommends that *all fats* be consumed sparingly. Take a look at the box above for a list of fatty foods. They're all good for you, they're full of essential vitamins and minerals, and they taste good. Just remember to eat them in moderation as part of your healthful diet.

> ### HEALTHY FATS
>
> Cold-pressed oils including canola, avocado, flaxseed, safflower, sunflower, corn, and walnut
>
> Extra-virgin olive oil
>
> Homemade salad dressings and mayonnaise
>
> Cold-water fish such as halibut, salmon, rainbow trout, sardines, tuna, mackerel, bluefish (high in omega-3 fatty acids and protein)
>
> Fresh, raw nuts (also contain a significant amount of protein)
>
> Fresh, certified organic raw butter
>
> Cheese and whole milk (also contain significant amounts of protein)

NUTRITIONAL SUPPLEMENTS: VITAMINS AND MINERALS

Unless you eat a 100 percent organic diet, get all the rest you need, have no stress in your life, and live on a pollution-free planet, then you probably need some sort of dietary supplementation. Pesticides, radiation, polluted water, smog, depleted soils, preservatives, antibiotics and hormones in the meat we eat, eating on the run, stress . . . all these things drain our bodies of essential nutrients. The average person's diet and lifestyle could use a little help!

THE GREAT DEBATE:
SYNTHETIC VS. NATURAL SUPPLEMENTS

Isolated and synthetic vitamins and minerals, whether mega-doses or minute amounts, do have their rightful place in the treatment of acute disease or severe nutritional deficiencies. But for those of us who are basically healthy and want to use supplements for the long haul to strengthen our immune system, help prevent disease, increase energy, and help keep the ravages of time at bay, I strongly recommend using natural, whole foods and herbs as supplements. Whole means just that: unfractionated, complete, and balanced, just as Mother Nature intended. I could never tell if the synthetic vitamins and isolated minerals that I took for years did any good. But I do know that I feel better, have more sustained energy and rarely get a cold or flu when I consistently consume whole food supplements. Synthetic laboratory-made supplements or nature-made? The choice is up to you.

I will not go into a detailed discussion of each and every isolated vitamin and mineral known and what condition they are good for. There are dozens of books available on the subject. Instead, I will offer a different approach to supplementation: whole food/herbal supplements. These supplements work slowly over a period of time to strengthen the body, add vitality, and give a long-lasting feeling of well-being. The alternative, megadoses of synthetic vitamins and isolated minerals, can produce a druglike effect or, at the very least, upset the body's delicate chemical balance. These supplement recipes are nontoxic and have no side effects except better health.

Many herbal companies offer herbal combination capsules (see resouces). I purchase most of my supplements from a wonderful herbalist, Jean Argus of Jean's Greens. She grinds fresh dried herbs and whole foods, then encapsulates them into 500 milligram veggie caps. She also will formulate a custom supplement for me if I feel I need to address a special health concern. Just make sure that the company you patronize uses primarily organically grown herbs and foods and has a rapid turnover rate. Natural products do lose their potency over time, especially if they are finely ground and encapsulated. The more processing a plant receives, the quicker it deteriorates.

The four recipes that follow are for basic herbal supplements that provide benefits for everyone. They are full of vitamins and minerals and cancer fighting antioxidants. A couple of them are quite tasty, too! Please try them, and as you gain more herbal knowledge, you can experiment, as I did, and learn to formulate your own combinations to suit your particular health needs. Here's to a long, vibrant life!

Note: All the herbs called for in the following recipes are in dried form and are available from better health food stores and the occasional "progressive" grocery store that has a health food and herb section. If your local stores don't carry them, you can order them from any of the mail-order suppliers listed in the resource section in the back of the book. These herbs have little or no known toxicity and are generally safe for consumption in the dosages suggested. If you are pregnant or using medication, check with your health professional before adding these supplements to your diet.

> Then God said, "Behold, I have given you every herb bearing seed which is upon the face of all the earth and every tree which has fruit bearing seed; it shall be food for you."
>
> Genesis 1:29

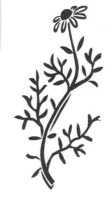

VITAMIN C TEA

I developed this delicious, earthy-tasting herb tea formula in the fall of 1996 just as the wild *Rosa rugosa* rosehips were beginning to dry on the bushes growing along the ocean down the street from my house. Rosehips are extremely high in vitamin C and bioflavonoids and are quite tart and refreshing. I drink this tea throughout the winter to help keep colds and flu at bay.

1 tablespoon (15 ml) rose hips

1 tablespoon (15 ml) dried raspberries or raspberry leaves

1 tablespoon (15 ml) chopped dandelion root

1 tablespoon (15 ml) dried strawberries or strawberry leaves

1 teaspoon (5 ml) cinnamon bark chips

½ teaspoon (2 ml) gingerroot

½ teaspoon (2 ml) stevia leaves (sweet herb)

Yield: approximately 8–12 cups of tea

To make: Combine all ingredients.

To use: Pour 1 cup (230 ml) of boiling water over 1 to 2 teaspoons (5 to 10 ml) of dried herb combination. Allow to steep at least 10 minutes, then strain. Add honey if desired.

For a stronger brew, bring 4 cups (1 liter) of water to boil. Reduce heat to barely a simmer and add 1½ tablespoons (22 ml) of dried herb combination. Allow to steep for 20 minutes, then strain.

Storage: Keep the remaining mixture in an airtight plastic bag or a dark glass jar with a tight-fitting lid. Store in a cool, dark, dry place.

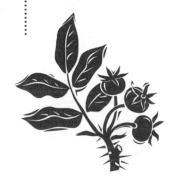

MY DAILY BREW

Break your morning coffee habit with this delicious tea. It's chock full of vitamins and minerals to get you started on the right foot (or left!).

- 2 tablespoons (30 ml) roasted, chopped chicory root
- 1 tablespoon (15 ml) raspberry leaves
- 1 tablespoon (15 ml) chopped dandelion root
- 1 tablespoon (15 ml) dried apples, finely chopped
- 1 tablespoon (15 ml) German chamomile flowers
- 1 tablespoon (15 ml) nettle leaves
- 1 tablespoon (15 ml) alfalfa grass
- 1 tablespoon (15 ml) oat straw
- 2 teaspoons (10 ml) dried cranberries (if unavailable, increase amount of rose hips by 2 teaspoons)
- 1 teaspoon (5 ml) rose hips
- 1 teaspoon (5 ml) cinnamon bark
- 1/2 teaspoon (2 ml) crushed or powdered nutmeg
- 1/2 teaspoon (2 ml) stevia leaves (sweet herb)

To make: Combine all ingredients.

To use: Pour 1 cup (230 ml) of boiling water over 1 to 2 teaspoons (5 to 10 ml) of dried herb combination. Allow to steep at least 10 minutes, then strain. Add honey if desired.

For a stronger brew, bring 4 cups of water to boil. Reduce heat to barely a simmer and add 1½ tablespoons (22 ml) of dried herb combination. Allow to steep for 20 minutes, then strain.

Storage: Keep the remaining mixture in an airtight plastic bag or a dark glass jar with a tight-fitting lid. Store in a cool, dark, dry place.

Yield: approximately 20–28 cups of tea

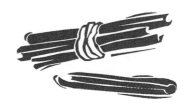

ALGAE: A NUTRITIONAL POWERHOUSE

There are more than forty thousand different species of algae. They include brown ocean kelp, which can grow to 100 feet long; red ocean algae, high in beta-carotene; and inedible protococcus, known fondly as "pond scum." Blue-green algae is the simplest of all the algae, and one that can have great benefits when taken in as a suppplement.

Blue-green algae is an excellent source of gamma linolenic acid (GLA), which can improve skin tone and mental clarity, aid in weight loss, and relieve symptoms of PMS and arthritis. It is also high in protein, beta-carotene, vitamins C, B complex, E, and K, essential fatty acids, trace minerals, enzymes, and chlorophyll. Chlorophyll is a photosynthetic pigment that aids in digestion, helps stop bacterial growth in wounds, and can eliminate bad breath and body odor.

I have been taking approximately 2 to 3 grams (under 1 ounce) of the aphanizomenon flos-aquae (AFA) form of blue-green algae (see resources) daily as a supplement for a couple of years now and have received many remarkable benefits, including the virtual elimination of terrible monthly menstrual cramps and PMS. It has also improved my normally clear skin and made it look spectacular. Many people mistake me for being ten years younger than I am. That's a definite plus!

Spirulina is another popular form of blue-green algae, but I have found the AFA form to work better for my particular health needs. Should you decide to try either algae, the benefits you receive may or may not be as dramatic as mine. But your overall health should improve provided you also eat a healthy diet and get plenty of exercise.

Capsules

For these two recipes, you'll either need a capsule filler (see box), or if you're very busy, have an herb supplier make the capsules for you. (Filling capsules by hand is time consuming.) Several of the companies listed in the resources section will gladly encapsulate your custom blend.

PLANT POWER CAPS

This formula contains vitamin B complex, vitamin C, beta-carotene, manganese, calcium, iron, magnesium, iodine, potassium, chlorophyll, and trace minerals.

2 tablespoons (30 ml) spirulina algae

1 tablespoon (15 ml) alfalfa grass

1 tablespoon (15 ml) dandelion leaves

1 tablespoon (15 ml) nettle leaves

1 tablespoon (15 ml) raspberry leaves

2 teaspoons (10 ml) rose hips

1 teaspoon (5 ml) kelp

1/2 teaspoon (2 ml) peppermint leaves

1/2 teaspoon (2 ml) cayenne pepper powder

Yield: Approximately fifty 500-milligram (size "00") capsules.

To make: Grind all ingredients except cayenne in a nut/seed grinder until completely powdered. Add the cayenne and combine gently to avoid eye and throat irritation. Make into capsules with the Cap-M-Quik capsule filler (see box).

Dosage: Up to six 500-milligram capsules daily. Start slowly and gradually build up to the level that makes you feel terrific.

MAKE YOUR OWN CAPSULES

If you want to make your own capsules, use the Cap-M-Quik encapsulating device. It's available in better health food stores or through Mountain Rose Herbs (see resources). It's a bit time consuming to use, but does allow you to make approximately fifty capsules at one time.

HAIR, SKIN, AND NAILS CAPSULES

Certain nutrients, in particular sulfur, silicon, and zinc, are vital to healthy hair, skin, and nails. They are essential in your daily diet and this capsule recipe includes those and many trace minerals as well.

2 tablespoons (30 ml) spirulina algae

1 tablespoon (15 ml) oat straw

1 tablespoon (15 ml) pumpkin seeds

1 tablespoon (15 ml) watercress

1 tablespoon (15 ml) kelp

2 teaspoons (15 ml) garlic granules

1 teaspoon (5 ml) horsetail herb

1/2 teaspoon (2 ml) cayenne pepper powder

To make: Grind all ingredients except cayenne in a nut/seed grinder until completely powdered. Add the cayenne and combine gently to avoid eye and throat irritation. Make into capsules with the Cap-M-Quik capsule filler (see box on the previous page).

Dosage: Up to six 500-milligram capsules daily. Start slowly and gradually build up to the level that makes you feel terrific.

Yield: Approximately fifty 500-milligram (size "00") capsules.

CAYENNE CAUTION

When working with cayenne pepper powder, it's a good idea to wear gloves to avoid skin irritation, and to keep your hands away from your eyes, nose, and mouth. Dust from the ground powder can also be dispersed into the air and cause eye and lung irritation, so mix the powder very gently.

WATER, WATER, WATER

Oxygen, water, food — three important ingredients for life. You can survive only five to twenty minutes without oxygen (depending on the circumstances), three to six days without water, and a few months without food if you absolutely have to.

If adequate water consumption is so important, then why do so many people drink so very little or none at all? Could it be that they don't consider it a vital nutrient, or that it has no flavor, no zing, no sweetness? We all seem to like a little "zip" in our mouths; that's why soda is so popular!

Water is extremely vital to your well-being. It facilitates virtually every function in your body, such as ridding it of waste products, regulating temperature, lubricating your joints, enabling digestion to take place, keeping your skin moist, and giving shape to your cells. Your blood is mostly water. In fact, your body is 70 to 75 percent water!

As to taste, if you don't like it, add some fresh squeezed lemon, lime, or orange juice or mix in a little bottled fruit juice. But by all means drink up! Depending on your body size, try to drink 2 to 2½ quarts (2 to 2½ liters) per day and more if you're very active. Fruit juice, herb teas, and juicy, raw fruits all count toward your daily water total. If that sounds like a lot, spread it out. Try to drink one cup an hour throughout the day. You'll know you're getting enough if your urine is pale yellow or clear (unless you're taking a lot of the B vitamins, which tend to color your urine bright yellow).

FOOT FACT

According to the makers of Dr. Scholl's foot care products, the average person walks 115,000 miles in a lifetime, equal to circling the globe nearly five times.

EXERCISE

Diet and exercise go hand in hand. Healthy food nourishes your body and plenty of exercise revs up your circulation, strengthens your muscles and bones, and makes you mentally more alert. It helps keep your blood pressure down and blood sugar level stable. Exercise oxygenates your blood and helps keep you limber. It can give you a more youthful, vibrant feeling and make you feel proud and confident. I could go on. If exercise can do all this, then why are you skimping on it?

There are two main types of exercise: aerobic and weight-training, and we need some of each to be fit.

Aerobic exercise is any exercise that causes the body to increase its intake of oxygen. Anything that causes your heart to beat faster and pump harder and make you break into a sweat is aerobic, including walking, jogging, running, rollerblading, and skiing. These exercises, done for thirty to forty minutes, are effective at burning fat and calories.

Find an aerobic activity you enjoy and do it regularly, three to five times per week, to reap the maximum benefits. If you're overweight, over thirty-five, have never exercised, or are on medication, see a health professional prior to beginning a new program.

Ironically, though aerobic exercise is a recommended part of a healthful living regimen, your feet can sometimes suffer. They're under so much added pressure from all your jumping, running, and walking that they easily succumb to injury if not properly shod and cared for. It's important to wear proper footwear for any type of exercise and attend to foot pain immediately.

Weight training involves performing a series of exercises while holding dumbbells or a weighted bar in your hands. Other weight-bearing exercises can be performed on various machines using cables or pulleys (such as those found in a gym) with the weight set according to your goals.

Training with weights tones and builds muscle size. Weight lifting also improves posture, strengthens bones, and enables you to perform more activities with ease. A well-muscled body also burns more calories per hour than a fatty physique.

After you've been regularly training for thirty minutes a day, twice a week, for a few months, you may notice that the scale has inched up a few pounds, but your clothes are looser. Muscle weighs more but takes up less space than fat, another benefit.

If the thought of exercising by yourself sounds boring, find a friend or join a gym. Find something you like to do and stick to it! You might even discover that you love it! I like to use exercise videotapes to get me moving in the winter. My favorite is a series called The FIRM. These videos offer a workout method called aerobic weight training. You work out aerobically while simultaneously lifting weights. This system produces the best results for me (see resources on page 177 for ordering information).

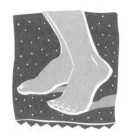

CHAPTER 2

MEET YOUR FEET: FOOT BASICS

If your feet could speak, what would they say?

"We're so cramped in these tight, pointy shoes, we're nearly numb," say the fashionable woman's feet.

"These shoes smell so bad it's embarrassing," say the feet of a young athlete.

"Our toes are ugly and deformed, we've got corns every-where, we ache, and you've painted our toenails a deep purple frost. Please don't show us in public!" say the feet of a hip young woman. (This is what *my* feet were saying in high school!)

"We can't breathe. Your designer Italian leather loafers and nylon socks are choking us. We look gorgeous but we're dying in here . . . please give us some air!" say the style-conscious attor-ney's feet.

If your feet could speak, they'd probably complain, and loudly. Our feet allow us to run, walk, jump, and skip, taking us where we need to go, often with grace and style. It's very difficult to get along without them. So what do we do to keep them in tip-top shape? Abuse them! Sometimes I think I should have titled this book *The Evils of Modern Footwear.*

You're going to hear me say this over and over again through-out this book: ill-fitting shoes are the source of most foot prob-lems. We stuff our feet into high heels or loafers with narrow toes or wrap them in nylon socks or stockings so they can't breathe. We buy shoes that are too small or inflexible and that irritate our feet. We also tend to wear shoes long past their designated life span until all the supportive cushioning is no longer able to do its job.

In addition to shoe abuse, our feet also suffer from lack of daily hygiene. How many people actually wash and scrub their feet (including the soles and between the toes), much less actually dry between the toes? When we bathe or shower most of us just assume that the soap and shampoo that runs onto our feet is sufficient. All of this neglect can lead to foot problems (see chapter 9, Common Foot Problems, Uncommon Remedies, for an alphabetical list of foot problems and their treatments).

Avoiding these problems starts with basic foot care, wearing appropriate shoes, and giving your feet the occasional pampering treatment, all of which I cover in later chapters. First, here are some basics on the structure and function of your feet.

YOUR AMAZING FOOT

A masterpiece of design, that's what your foot is. Your complex, small foot contains some 26 bones (both feet contain a quarter of the bones in your entire body), 33 joints, and 112 ligaments, and a complicated network of blood vessels, tendons, and nerves. All of these interworking parts enable you to move gracefully, with balance and speed if you so wish. The heel pad and arches of your foot act as shock absorbers, cushioning blows and jolts that occur with every step.

Basic daily living, doing your household chores, walking around your office or in the grocery store, or just walking the dog, exerts several hundred tons of pressure on your feet over the course of the day. Feet experience more wear and tear in a

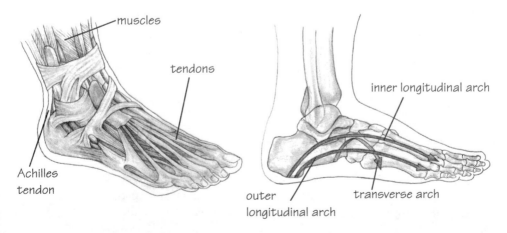

muscles

tendons

Achilles
tendon

inner longitudinal arch

outer
longitudinal arch

transverse arch

lifetime than any other body part, and thus are more prone to injury. Of all the physical ailments people have, foot problems may be the most common.

Foot shape, size, arch height, and length of toes vary from person to person. The feet you have are an inherited combination from your parents, which may predispose you to several foot problems, including bunions, high arches, or Morton's foot.

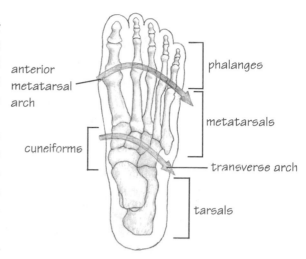

phalanges

metatarsals

transverse arch

tarsals

anterior metatarsal arch

cuneiforms

Toenails

Toenails are composed of the same protein as your skin and hair, keratin. They just happen to have a harder composition. Their purpose is to protect the ends of your toes and the bones and nerves lying underneath. Toenails grow approximately ¹⁄₁₆ inch to ⅛ inch (1.6 mm to 3 mm) per month, slower than fingernails.

Your toenails can suffer a variety of disorders caused by injury, poor hygiene, poor circulation, or disease, such as bruises, tears, thick nails, ingrown nails, fungus, club nail, discoloration, brittleness, and curved growth. The elderly are especially susceptable to toenail problems due to failing eyesight and lack of strength to properly cut their nails, or simply because they can't bend over to do proper maintenance.

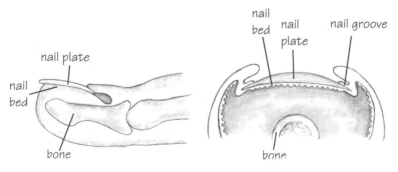

nail plate

nail bed

bone

nail bed

nail plate

nail groove

bone

FOOT CARE BASICS

Treat your feet with tender loving care and they'll reward you with years of diligent, pain-free service. Just follow these simple guidelines for healthy, happy feet.

- ◆ Wash your feet daily. Make sure to get between the toes and under the nails.
- ◆ Completely dry your feet after bathing. Make sure to get between the toes when drying, too. Damp feet provide a breeding ground for bacteria and odor.
- ◆ To help prevent dry, cracked foot skin, massage a good thick lotion into your feet before you dress and again before you go to bed.
- ◆ Add a little foot powder to your shoes each day to help absorb perspiration.
- ◆ Wear fresh socks or hosiery daily.
- ◆ Cut your toenails straight across to help avoid ingrown toenails. Afterwards, smooth nail edges with an emery board or nail file.
- ◆ Inspect your feet daily for blisters, corns, calluses, swelling or other problems and treat accordingly. An ounce of prevention is worth a pound of cure.
- ◆ Give your shoes a rest. Alternating pairs allows shoes to completely dry out and gives the padding time to return to its normal shape. This makes shoes last longer and keeps your feet healthier.
- ◆ Give yourself a weekly "feet treat." Massage your feet with warmed oil mixed with a few drops of essential oil of lavender, eucalyptus, or peppermint to de-stress and relax your sore feet. I can hear them now: "Ahhhhh, that feels good!"
- ◆ If you're overweight, lose some pounds. Excess weight adds enormous pressure to your already stressed feet.

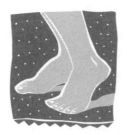

CHAPTER 3

INGREDIENTS, SUPPLIES, AND TOOLS OF THE TRADE

Many of my friends ask me to custom make herbal creams, salves, lotions, or scrubs for them because they assume that making your own personal care products is a complicated and time consuming task. As with anything in life, the first attempt at learning something new takes a bit of time, but with just a little practice, it can become second nature. Once you learn the basics of creating herbal products at home, you'll be hooked! If you have rudimentary cooking skills, then you're all set.

This chapter describes the ingredients and equipment necessary to create the herbal recipes found throughout this book. It also covers the basic foot care treatment supplies that are used for specific problems in chapter 9. The ingredients that include botanical names are those particular varieties that I recommend using in my recipes.

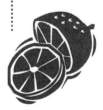

WHEN IN DOUBT, CHECK IT OUT

Anytime you use essential oils and herbs, it's a good idea to follow general safety precautions (see boxes on the next two pages for how to do patch tests). Years ago, when I was but a novice when it came to using herbs for health and beauty, I decided to make a bath oil using essential oil of lemon. I mixed my tablespoon of almond oil and a few drops of lovely, refreshing essential oil of lemon and poured it into my running bath water, anticipating a refreshing, skin tingling bath. Ahhh, I could hardly wait!

I slipped right in. It felt and smelled so good . . . for the first three minutes, that is. In less than six to seven minutes, my skin-tingling bath had turned into a red, rashy, skin-burning affair that made me feel like I'd just sat down on a hill of fire ants! It was horrible! I immediately rinsed off and doused myself with a bottle of cold aloe vera gel that I always keep in the refrigerator. It helped a little, but I continued to itch and burn for the rest of the evening.

The moral of the story is, just because it's all natural doesn't mean it can't bother you! Everyone is allergic to something at some point in their lives, whether synthetic or natural. When making any natural personal care recipe, never use a new ingredient without first doing a patch test, especially if the ingredient is an unfamiliar essential oil or herbal extract.

Some essential oils that may be particularly irritating to the skin include allspice, bitter almond, camphor, cinnamon, clove, fir needle, grapefruit, lemon, lemongrass, lime, orange, peppermint, pine, sage, and wintergreen. The citrus oils can also cause photosensitivity, so stay out of the sun if these have been applied to your skin.

Aura Cacia (see resources) recommends avoiding the following essential oils during pregnancy: bitter almond, basil, clary sage, clove bud, sweet fennel, juniper berry, marjoram, myrrh, peppermint, rose, rosemary, sage, thyme, and wintergreen.

Some herbs and ingredients may be irritating to the skin. These include allspice, aloe vera, benzoin tincture, chamomile, cocoa butter, cornstarch, glycerine, grapefruit peel and juice, juniper, lanolin, lemon peel and juice, lime peel and juice, orange peel and juice, peppermint, pine needles, and wintergreen.

HOW TO DO A PATCH TEST WITH HERBS

In a small bowl, combine $1/2$ teaspoon (2 ml) of the fresh or dried chopped herb in question with 1 teaspoon (5 ml) or so of boiling water. Let the herb absorb the water for a few minutes. Apply a dab of the herb to the inside of your upper arm or wrist area; cover with an adhesive strip and leave in place 12 to 24 hours. If no irritation develops the herb is generally safe to use.

ALCOHOL

Alcohol is used by herbalists as a menstruum (solvent) for extracting the healing elements from herbs. It dissolves and extracts resins, essential oils, fats, alkaloids, waxes, and other plant constituents. Alcohol is an excellent preservative: alcohol-based herbal extract preparations will last almost indefinitely, while water-based solutions will decompose in a matter of days.

ETHYL ALCOHOL (GRAIN ALCOHOL)

Common Names: Vodka, brandy, gin, rum, whiskey, and so forth.

Description: Derived from the fermentation of grains.

Uses: Commonly used for consumption in alcoholic beverages. I use it for making herbal extracts (tinctures) to take internally for tonic and medicinal purposes. I also use it to make herbal liniments, which are applied externally to soothe and aid in healing a number of skin problems.

Where to obtain: Must be over age 21 to legally purchase in a liquor store.

BASE OILS

Base oils are, as their name implies, a base to which essential oils and herbs are added when making herbal-infused oil, lotion, or cream. They can also be used on their own as bath oils, hair and skin conditioners, and great makeup removing solvents.

The best oils to purchase for cosmetic use are cold-pressed or expeller–pressed oils (rather than oils refined by chemical or heat extraction), since they are the highest quality and receive the least processing. For olive oil, the term "extra-virgin" also refers to the first pressing of the fruit. Subsequent pressings result in gradually lower quality oil.

If possible, take a whiff of any oil before you buy it. It should have only a trace of fragrance, if any at all. If it smells strong or off, then it's probably old. Don't buy it or, if you've purchased it from a mail-order supplier, return it and try again.

> **HOW TO DO AN ESSENTIAL OIL PATCH TEST**
>
> Combine 1 or 2 drops of the essential oil in question with 1 teaspoon (5 ml) base oil in a small bowl. Apply a dab on your wrist, inside your upper arm, behind your ear, or behind your knee, and wait 12 to 24 hours. If no irritation develops, it is generally safe to use the essential oil.

In a few places throughout this book I use the words *slip* or *slide* to describe the characteristic of an oil. These terms refer to the way an oil or a product glides onto the skin. When I say that an oil *slides well* or has a *nice slip,* I mean that it goes on effortlessly. An oil with this property is not too thick for use as a massage oil. My favorite oils for massage are almond and soybean. They have a thinner texture than other oils. You may like jojoba or olive because they have a thicker texture. The following are some of my favorite base oils and most are easy to find.

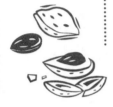

ALMOND OIL
Common Name: Sweet almond oil
Description: The oil is derived from the ripened, pressed kernel of the fruit stone. It's edible, nontoxic, and is generally clear to very pale yellow in color with little to slightly nutty fragrance.
Uses: A classic beauty oil that has a medium weight and penetrates and pampers the skin wonderfully, almond oil is used in the manufacture of better creams, lotions, massage oils, lip balms, and facial cleansers. Most of the almond oil available is expeller-pressed, or cosmetic grade, but food-grade oil is occasionally available in bulk; either is fine for the recipes in this book. Store your almond oil in the refrigerator to prevent it from going rancid.

In addition to almond oil, I use ground almonds in scrub mixtures to help slough away and relieve dry skin. To make, simply put a handful of raw almonds in a nut/seed grinder or coffee grinder or blender and grind until the consistency of parmesan cheese.
Where to obtain: Cosmetic-grade almond oil and raw almonds are available in health food stores and through mail-order catalogs.

CASTOR OIL
Common Names: Castor oil plant, Palma Christi, Mexico seed
Description: The pressed seeds yield a very shiny, thick oil that is nontoxic unless ingested in large amounts. The seeds are toxic and can be fatal.
Uses: I like to use this thick, shiny oil as a base when making foot and hand massage oils and when I want a lip balm with real

staying power. I find it too thick to use as an overall massage oil because it doesn't slide very well.

"Turkey Red" oil is a form of castor oil that has sulfuric acid added to it to make it dissolve in water. Turkey red oil is completely water soluble and thus makes a great bath oil base. It should be stored in the refrigerator.

Where to obtain: Most health food stores and some drugstores carry castor oil. Try to find the odorless and tasteless form. Turkey Red oil is usually available only through mail-order suppliers.

JOJOBA OIL

Common Names: Jojoba, goat nut, wax plant

Description: Top quality jojoba oil is derived from the cold-pressed, organically grown seeds of this evergreen desert shrub. The seeds yield a clear to very pale yellow, odorless liquid wax (it is technically not an oil). A little goes a long way, which is a good thing, because jojoba oil is very expensive compared to the other base oils. Jojoba oil has a long shelf life and needs no refrigeration. It will not turn rancid.

Uses: This is one of my favorite oils because it's rich, thick, and good for winter-dry skin. It's edible, nontoxic, and generally nonirritating and it makes a superb skin conditioner.

Where to obtain: Health food stores and mail-order companies usually carry the oil.

OLIVE OIL

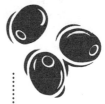

Common Names: Olive or Oliva

Description: Ripe, black olive fruits are pressed for olive oil. It can range in color from very pale green-gold to dark, almost cloudy green. Has a distinctive "olive" flavor, depending on the degree of processing and type of olive tree. Extra-virgin, cold-pressed olive oil is recommended, as it has had the least amount of processing. Olive oil should be refrigerated unless used within thirty days. It will eventually turn rancid.

Uses: It is used cosmetically as a base for herbal creams, massage and solar infused oils, lotions, hair conditioners, and soap.

Where to obtain: Most grocery and health food stores carry the top quality oil. It's also available through mail-order suppliers.

SOYBEAN OIL

Common Name: Soybean

Description: Soybean oil is valued as a food and cosmetic ingredient. It is almost always refined and is pale yellow in color, with a bland flavor.

Uses: I use soybean oil when I make massage oil products. I like its slip and the way it penetrates and softens the skin without leaving an oily residue (if you don't use too much). I also use it in light skin creams and lotions. Though it is edible, I don't use it for cooking because I prefer a cold-pressed oil to a highly refined one.

If you're on a tight budget, this is the oil to use. It's inexpensive, easy to find, and can be used in almost every foot care recipe in this book that calls for oil. It's not my number one choice, but it will work in a pinch.

Where to obtain: Any grocery store should carry soybean oil. Sometimes the front label will say "vegetable oil"; check the ingredient label and it will probably say "100 percent soybean oil." Some health food stores and mail-order suppliers carry it, but not many do, since it's not a specialty oil and is rarely found in cold-pressed form.

"NEAT" ESSENTIAL OILS

Essential oils are so highly concentrated that very few may be used "neat" (undiluted) on the skin. The exceptions are lavender, tea tree, German chamomile, rose, sandalwood, and geranium.

ESSENTIAL OILS

I refer to essential oils as the "soul of the plant." They are the plant's life force, a gift from Mother Nature, extracted and bottled for our help in healing.

Essential oils are present in various plant parts and are usually extracted by steam distillation, with the exception of citrus oils, which are generally cold-pressed from the rind. They are found in the leaves and twigs of peppermint and spearmint, the flowers of lavender and rose, the bark of the cinnamon tree, the flower buds of the clove tree, the wood of cedar, the roots of vetiver and ginger, and the seeds of coriander and cardamom. The resins of some trees and bushes yield such essential oils as myrrh and frankincense, while the needles of fir and pine produce lovely, fresh, clean "holiday" oils.

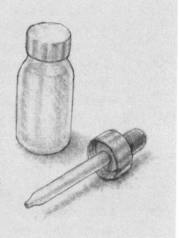
Essential oils are highly concentrated and must be used with caution. One precious drop of essential oil is the approximate equivalent of one teaspoon of the *dried* herb or spice. Unlike fatty vegetable oils, they are not prone to rancidity. They do not dissolve in water and only a little bit in vinegar. They *do* mix very well in vegetable, nut, and seed base oils such as jojoba, olive, soybean, and castor, and they dissolve relatively well in alcohol.

Always educate yourself about the properties and contraindications surrounding each essential oil before you use it. Dilute in a base oil before use, unless you are very familiar with a particular oil and have used it neat before. Store essential oils in a dark, dry, cool place. They can retain their healing properties for years if stored properly. Because they can be harmful if ingested, it is also important to store them out of reach of children and pets.

CAMPHOR

Common Names: Camphor tree, laurel camphor

Description: The clear to yellow essential oil and solid white crystals are derived from the distillation of roots or wood from a twenty-five to fifty year old tree.

Uses: Camphor essential oil is very cooling to the skin, helps relieve itching, and acts as a natural preservative. In other countries, camphor essential oil and crystals are used as an antiseptic and anthelmintic (rids body of worms). Camphor is known as "the original mothball."

I like to use camphor essential oil mixed with peppermint essential oil in cooling foot sprays and creams to soothe tired, sore, hot feet. It is also good combined with eucalyptus, clove, peppermint, and wintergreen essential oils and made into a salve for chest colds.

Where to obtain: Some pharmacies carry it, but check the label, as it may be synthetic. The real camphor essential oil is available from better health food stores and the crystals are usually mail-order only.

CHAMOMILE, GERMAN (MATRICARIA RECUTITA)

Common Names: Blue chamomile, wild chamomile, sweet false chamomile

Description: An annual, self-seeding herb with small, daisy-like flowers. The essential oil is a deep blue color, which comes from the component azulene that is formed during the distillation process.

Uses: Chamomile essential oil has anti-inflammatory and anti-fungal properties and helps speed wound healing. The flowers produce a pale yellow tea that is calming, relaxing, and soothing to jangled nerves and upset stomachs. A cold or cool foot bath of pure infusion of chamomile makes a great treatment for odoriferous and itchy, rashy feet.

I like to use the fresh flowers from my garden for making a solar infused herbal oil and teas. The dried, ground herb is great in powders and facial scrubs and the beautiful, blue oil I use to treat acne pimples, open sores, and poison ivy. The essential oil is one of the few oils that can be used neat on the skin to calm any irritation and reddening. It works like a charm!

Where to obtain: Both the dried herb and essential oil are available in better health food stores, herb shops, and mail-order supply houses. The essential oil is on the expensive side, but it's worth every dollar!

> Smell is a potent wizard that transplants us across thousands of miles and all the years we have lived.
>
> Helen Keller

CLARY SAGE (SALVIA SCLAREA)

Description: Clary sage is a biennial herb with serrated oval leaves, producing small purple, pink, or white flowers on squarish stems. The entire plant (as well as the essential oil) smells balsamlike.

Uses: This essential oil is used as a fixative in the making of perfumes, an antidepressant, a flavoring, a cosmetic fragrance, and a powerful relaxant. It is excellent to use in a soothing, de-stressing footbath at the end of the day.

Where to obtain: Most good health food stores and herb shops carry this popular oil, as do mail-order suppliers.

CLOVE

Common Name: Clove

Description: Dried cloves are the unripened flower buds of the plant that are dried in the sun until they turn brown. The essential oil is distilled from the fresh leaves and flower buds and is warming and spicy and yellow to pale yellow-brown to dark brown in color.

Uses: Clove oil is one of the most powerful germicidal agents in the plant kingdom, as well as being a potent antiseptic and stimulant. It is used to treat indigestion, nausea, vomiting, ringworm, athlete's foot, toothache, and bad breath.

I use the essential oil in warming, spicy massage oils, and salves for chest colds. A drop or two is great for an occasional toothache, too. Powdered cloves can add a bit of spice and anti-septic quality to foot powder and a nice scent to facial scrubs.

Where to obtain: Clove powder can be purchased in your grocery store and some herb shops and health food stores. Buy the essential oil in health food stores and through mail-order catalogs.

EUCALYPTUS

Common Names: Eucalyptus, blue gum tree

Description: The essential oil is pale green to pale yellow and derived from mature leaves and twigs.

Uses: The uses are many for this pleasant-smelling, refreshing essential oil. It is used in cough drops, vapor rubs for colds and flu to help ease breathing and chest congestion, and inhalation steams to help clear bronchial tubes.

I use it in a cooling antiseptic and deodorant footbath and powder. It leaves your feet feeling quite refreshed. It's great for deodorizing a stuffy room, too.

Where to obtain: Health food stores and mail-order catalogs.

GERANIUM *(PELARGONIUM GRAVEOLENS)*
Common Name: Scented rose geranium
Description: The scented geranium (not the common decorative nursery geranium) has rose/peppermint scented leaves. They refresh the air when you brush up against them. The essential oil, distilled from the leaves and twigs, is clear to very pale green.
Uses: I use this antiseptic and antifungal essential oil because I love the fragrance. The essential oil is also nice when added to a massage oil base and mixed with lavender, rose, and spearmint essential oils. If you want to really pamper yourself, make a body cream with geranium, rose, and lavender essential oils. Geranium essential oil added to a footbath helps heal poison ivy, athlete's foot, and skin sores. It's also good added to a refreshing, deodorizing foot spray.
Where to obtain: Grow a plant or two around the house to bask in their fragrance. Buy the essential oil from health food stores or through mail-order catalogs.

LAVENDER *(LAVANDULA ANGUSTIFOLIA)*
Common Name: Lavender
Description: The plant is shrubby, producing highly fragrant purple flowers. The essential oil is produced from steam-distilled flowers and is clear to yellowish-green in color.
Uses: This gentle yet powerful essential oil is a jack-of-all-trades. I use it to make soothing lotions and creams for face and body. It can be used neat on pimples and infections and on burns to help prevent scarring. The dried, powdered flowers make a fragrant foot powder when mixed with cornstarch. Lavender is highly antiseptic, very calming for nervous tension, and excellent for acne, eczema, and psoriasis.
Where to obtain: Plant a few simply to enjoy for their beauty and fragrance, if not to harvest for making an infused oil. The essential oil and dried herb can be purchased at health food stores and herb shops and through mail-order catalogs.

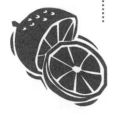

ORANGE, SWEET
Common Name: Sweet orange
Description: Sweet orange essential oil is cold-pressed from the rind and is pale orange to orange in color, wonderfully fragrant, and fresh smelling. It is highly volatile.

Uses: I use sweet orange essential oil as an uplifting, refreshing fragrance in lotions, creams, and foot scrubs. Orange flower water is distilled from the flowers and is great for sensitive, dry skin with broken capillaries. The essential oil is terrific in men's powders and aftershaves. For a masculine scent, mix it with essential oil of lime, peppermint, and earthy oils such as clove and cinnamon. It has astringent qualities and is good blended with alcohol and used as a deodorizing foot spray. Dried orange peel can be finely ground and used in foot and body scrubs.

Where to obtain: Sweet orange essential oil is available in cooking stores, health food stores, and through mail order.

PEPPERMINT *(MENTHA X PIPERITA)*

Common Names: Brandy mint, lamb mint, mint

Description: Peppermint essential oil is derived from distilled leaves and stems and is clear to pale green-yellow in color. I have purchased peppermint essential oil only to be disappointed that it smelled like pennyroyal and mint combined. Ask the supplier if it really smells truly minty, like candy or sweeter. Though more expensive than other varieties, French peppermint oil seems to be of higher quality than most, with a true minty fragrance and sharp bite. Aura Cacia (see resources) carries a superior peppermint essential oil.

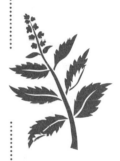

Uses: The high percentage of menthol in peppermint is responsible for its praised medicinal qualities. The tea is used as a cure for indigestion and gas, a mouthwash, facial astringent for normal-to-oily skin, and makes a refreshing foot bath for smelly, hot feet. I use the oil as a breath freshener and to add antiseptic, antiviral, astringent, and cooling properties to lotions, foot creams, and scrubs. The powdered leaves are a nice addition to foot and body powders.

Where to obtain: By all means grow a patch, just don't let it take over your whole garden! The essential oil and dried herb is available in health food stores, herb shops, and through mail order.

ROSEMARY *(ROSMARINUS OFFICINALIS)*

Common Name: Rosemary

Description: The essential oil is derived from distillation of the plant's resinous leaves and is usually clear to pale yellow in color.

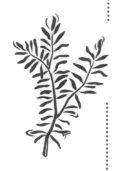

Uses: Rosemary essential oil can be used alone or in combination with thyme oil and sage tea in a deodorizing footbath that also helps relieve aching feet.

I like to add the dried herb to bath bags, mixed with a few drops of essential oil and a handful of oatmeal for a softening and stimulating bath. Rosemary essential oil makes a refreshing, antiseptic, deodorizing, antibacterial, and antifungal foot spray if mixed with tea tree essential oil and stored in the refrigerator to keep cool.

Where to obtain: Purchase the herb and essential oil from health food stores, herb shops, and through mail-order suppliers.The herb can be grown in a pot or your garden, depending on climate, and dried for teas and bathing/culinary uses.

ROSE OTTO/ATTAR *(ROSA X DAMASCENA* OR *ROSA X CENTIFOLIA)*

Common Name: Damask rose

Description: Both rose otto and rose attar come from the shrubby damask rose, which is cultivated for its precious essential oil in Bulgaria, Southern France, Russia, and Turkey; it grows wild throughout the Northern Hemisphere. Rose otto differs from rose absolute in that it is steam-distilled rather than being solvent extracted. Rose otto is preferred for aromatherapy use.

This is one of the most sought-after and expensive perfume materials in the world. One ounce (28 g) can cost upward of five hundred dollars (retail). It can be purchased in minute amounts. The essential oil is clear to yellow in color and semisolid at a cool room temperature. It has a beautiful floral, mildly spicy, romantic, haunting fragrance. If you want to substitute, geranium essential oil will work in its place.

Uses: I use the essential oil in my personal perfume, to calm my nerves, scent face and body creams, and make a mildly astringent rose water for my skin. The flowers are also dried for potpourri or powdered for body and foot powders. Rose water is a by-product of essential oil manufacture and is used in making creams and facial toners.

Where to obtain: Be careful where you purchase this essential oil, as much of the oil on the market is diluted with other essential oils or alcohol or is synthetic. Once you have smelled the real thing, you can usually sniff out a fake in a second! I never buy rose oil from health food or herb stores. They generally don't stock it anyway because of the expense. I purchase through the mail-order suppliers listed in the resource section.

SPEARMINT (MENTHA X SPICATA)

Common Names: Lamb mint, mint, Our Lady's mint

Description: Spearmint is very similar to peppermint, though it is not as high in menthol content and has a fresher, sweeter, and less harsh fragrance. The essential oil is distilled from leaves and stems and is clear to very pale green in color.

Uses: Use the same as peppermint oil. I like to mix peppermint, spearmint, and orange essential oils into a body or foot lotion and scrub. The combination is very refreshing and deodorizing. The essential oil makes great breath mint drops. It can also be used as a freshening room spray. Mixed with peppermint oil and vodka or isopropyl alcohol, it makes a cooling leg and foot spray.

Where to obtain: The herb and essential oil can be purchased from herb and health food shops or mail order. Try growing a small patch.

TEA TREE

Common Name: Tea tree

Description: The essential oil is derived from distillation of the tree's leaves and is yellowish in color. It has a strong medicinal, camphorlike, piney fragrance.

Uses: Tea tree essential oil could be described as nature's first aid kit in a bottle. It is powerful as an antifungal, germicidal, and antiseptic and can be used neat on pimples, cuts, bug bites, toothache, bleeding gums, ringworm, athlete's foot, and warts. Tea tree essential oil does not generally irritate skin tissue and stimulates rapid healing.

I use it when making foot powders, liniments, and salves to treat athlete's foot, toenail fungus, and poison ivy. Used in lip balms, it helps heal cold sores. I gargle with hot water, a pinch of cayenne, and a drop or two of tea tree essential oil if I feel a sore throat coming on and inhale for a stuffy nose.

Where to obtain: The oil can be purchased in herb and health food shops and through mail order.

THYME, RED *(THYMUS VULGARIS* **OR** *THYMUS ZYGIS)*
Common Names: Common thyme, garden thyme
Description: This powerful antibacterial and antiseptic essential oil is distilled from the leaves and flowers.
Uses: I like to add the oil to powders and salves to combat foot odor, athlete's foot, ulcers, psoriasis, and eczema. Place the dried herb into a bath bag with rosemary, oatmeal, and tea tree essential oil to help heal poison ivy and itchy, rashy skin.
Where to obtain: Purchase dried herb and essential oil in herb shops and health food stores and through mail order. Grow in your garden if you can. It's stimulating to sniff a fresh sprig.

CLAYS

Clay has been used cosmetically and therapeutically for centuries in mud baths, face and body packs, ceremonial rituals, hair cleansing and conditioning treatments, drawing poultices for increasing local circulation, and exfoliation of dead surface skin.

Excavated in mines throughout France and parts of Europe and North America, clay is rich in minerals derived from plants, animals, water, soil, rocks, and volcanic ash that have been compounded and slowly ground into extremely fine particles. These particles have been deposited by rivers and streams in large masses, usually in the banks of lakes and rivers or near underground water channels.

As the clay is formed it picks up various trace minerals that impart earthy colors such as green, white, yellow, red, brown, black, and gray. Each color contains different concentrations of minerals. Green is high in calcium, magnesium, potassium, sodium, iron, silica, and plant materials. Yellow clay contains sulphur; red clay contains iron; brown and black have iron, zinc, and sulphur; and white contains zinc, silica, calcium, and magnesium.

When liquid is added to dehydrated, powdered clay, the clay becomes a soft, pliable mass that can be molded into any shape or merely spread as a paste. This property, in addition to the mineral richness, makes it a terrific ingredient to use when thickening salves, making masks and scrubs, and turning your bath water into a "mineral spa." The following three varieties of clay are my favorites and are easy to find. I always purchase clay in powdered form, not wet, unless it's in a prepared formula.

BENTONITE CLAY

Description: The name comes from Benton, Montana. It is an off-white to gray volcanic ash that occurs in the midwestern United States and Canada. It has a medium-fine texture. When mixed with water, bentonite clay has a very slippery, almost gel-like consistency. It can be lumpy and a bit grainier than other clays.

Uses: It is widely used in commercially prepared facial makeup, masks, and as a thickener. I use it to treat pimples, as a tightening facial mask, and to help treat poison ivy. It can also be used to make a mineral-rich foot pack to help heal athlete's foot and sores. Bentonite clay is good for all skin types except sensitive.

Where to obtain: I can usually find this clay only through mail-order suppliers.

GREEN CLAY

Common Names: French green clay or food grade green clay

Description: Green clay is light to dark sage green in color with a medium-fine texture.

Uses: Although green clay is good for all skin types, it is especially good for oily skin and for healing conditions that need drawing, astringency, sloughing, and circulation stimulation such as acne, eczema, psoriasis, shingles, hemorrhoids, devitalized, wrinkled skin, and dry, cracked skin on legs and feet.

Where to obtain: Again, I can rarely find this clay in health food stores or herb shops and must resort to mail order.

WHITE COSMETIC CLAY

Common names: Fine white clay, china clay, kaolin

Description: This clay is off-white to cream in color with a very fine texture; it is naturally absorbent.

Uses: White cosmetic clay is used commercially in face and body powders, liquid powders, and makeup. It is recommended for all skin types, especially sensitive and dry. I use white cosmetic clay blended with cornstarch and arrowroot and sometimes finely ground rose, lavender, or German chamomile flowers and spices to make a nice body or foot powder. Tea tree essential oil can be added to treat athlete's foot. Essential oils of peppermint and eucalyptus are good added to it to deodorize and cool.

Where to obtain: A few herb shops and health food stores carry white clay, but I usually order through mail-order suppliers.

HERBS

As recently as the nineteenth century, herbs were the primary source of medicine for both the Native Americans and the "civilized" folk. Most people knew how to use the local plants to concoct remedies to relieve common ailments. It's really too bad that this practice has fallen by the wayside.

Learning about herbs and their history, uses, and properties can be fascinating. Herbalism is enjoying a resurgence in popularity today and many, many new products are popping up on the market touting the benefits of the herbs they contain. I think it wise to educate yourself on at least the most commonly used healing herbs. Below is a listing and description of the herbs I use most in the personal care products I create.

> He causeth the grass to grow for the cattle and herbs for the service of humanity.
>
> Psalm 104:14

CALENDULA *(CALENDULA OFFICINALIS)*
Common Name: Pot marigold
Description: The lovely calendula has antispasmodic, antifungal, antiseptic, and antibacterial properties.
Uses: Fresh, golden-orange infused calendula flower oil helps heal cuts, bruises, scrapes, rashes, and sore muscles. Made into a salve or cream it can be used to treat athlete's foot when combined with lavender, tea tree, and thyme essential oils.

Calendula, black walnut, and goldenseal tincture combined with tea tree essential oil is an excellent formula to get rid of toenail fungus and ringworm. Dried calendula blossoms can be ground into a powder and combined with ground German chamomile, cornstarch, and white cosmetic clay for a soothing, mild baby powder or children's foot powder. The sticky sap is said to remove warts when applied daily for several months.
Where to obtain: Please try to grow a patch and make your own infused oil. (See the recipe for Calendula Blossom Oil on page 132.) You'll save money this way since calendula oil is on the expensive side. The dried petals and infused oil are available at better health food stores and herb shops and always through mail-order sources.

CAYENNE PEPPER

Common Names: Capsicum, chili pepper, Spanish pepper, African bird pepper

Description: The active ingredient is a substance called *capsaicin,* which acts as a powerful analgesic, stimulant, antibacterial, and antiviral agent. Cayenne gets its name from the Greek word meaning "to bite," and indeed it does!

Uses: Cayenne can be incorporated into an ointment to be applied to painful joints, cuts, and bruises to stimulate circulation and healing. The powder can be sprinkled into socks to warm the feet.

Caution: Cayenne pepper is very, very hot and spicy! If ingesting, use it sparingly at first until your taste buds adjust to the heat. Keep away from eyes and mucous membranes.

Where to obtain: The best source for hot and effective dried peppers and tinctures is The American Botanical Pharmacy (see resources). If you can find fresh habañero peppers in the grocery store, then make your own fresh tincture.

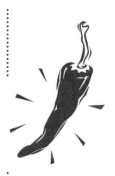

CHAMOMILE, GERMAN (See description under Essential Oils.)

CHAPARRAL *(LARREA TRIDENTATA)*

Common Names: Stinkweed, creosote bush, greasewood

Description: This herb's antiseptic and antibiotic properties come from the leaflets and twigs. It tastes terrible. It's very bitter, like tar, and stinks to boot! Thus the name.

Uses: Chaparral is excellent to use as a tea for a cavity preventative mouthwash, if you can stand the taste! It is also good to use in powdered form blended with cornstarch and baking soda for a foot powder to help heal athlete's foot and kill infection.

Where to obtain: Harvest from the wild if you can or order through mail order.

CLARY SAGE (See description under Essential Oils.)

CLOVE (See description under Essential Oils.)

COMFREY *(SYMPHYTUM OFFICINALE)*

Common Names: Gum plant, knitbone, boneset, healing herb, slippery root

Description: The leaves and especially the root produce a soothing mucilage when barely simmered in water (not boiled). The main healing compound in comfrey is *allantoin,* which promotes new cell and tissue growth.

Uses: Comfrey has been used for centuries as a popular healing herb. The mucilage is soothing to cuts, bruises, dry skin, ulcers, hot, itchy feet, and athlete's foot. The slimy goo produced from the roots, when made into a lotion, is so very gentle it's recommended for healing children's "boo-boos." I like to make a cream combining comfrey with plantain and vegetable shortening and use this on dry legs and cracked feet, hands, and nails. It soaks right in and is nongreasy.

Where to obtain: Grow a few plants if you can in an area where they won't invade your other garden herbs. The dried root and leaf is carried in most herb shops, health food stores, and via mail order.

GARLIC

Common Names: Garlic, clove garlic, stinking rose

Description: A perennial or biennial herb with an edible bulb consisting of ten to twenty cloves covered in thin, white papery skins. The green stems and white to lavender flowers are edible also. The main ingredient in garlic that gives it its medicinal quality and odor is *allicin.*

Uses: Garlic has been used for centuries as a germ killer, antiseptic, antibiotic, antiviral, anthelmintic (rids body of worms), and killer of fungi and yeasts, such as those responsible for athlete's foot. Garlic is high in sulfur, a necessary mineral promoting hair, skin, and nail health.

Caution: Be careful when applying raw garlic to your skin, as it is sometimes irritating.

Where to obtain: Organically grown garlic is available from health food stores, and ordinary garlic can be purchased from your regular grocery store.

GOLDENSEAL *(HYDRASTIS CANADENSIS)*

Common Names: Yellow root, Indian turmeric, jaundice root, golden root

Description: Goldenseal is cultivated for its roots and is rapidly being depleted in the wild by unethical harvesters. It tends to be expensive due to this overharvesting. The roots must be at least four years old to be harvested. An equally effective substitute is Oregon grape root, sometimes called western goldenseal, which is abundantly available and less expensive.

Uses: The root, when made into a tea, yields a very bitter, astringent-tasting liquid, which can be used as a gargle for sore throat or a skin wash for sores and acne. Goldenseal is a potent antibiotic and antiseptic and when made into a tincture is a good treatment for athlete's foot. A salve made from the yellow roots acts as a soothing, healing, moisturizing agent when applied to infected wounds, cuts, and insect bites.

Where to obtain: I discourage anyone from harvesting this herb, because of its endangerment. Plant seeds if you wish to encourage new plants, but don't wildcraft. Better herb shops and mail-order suppliers always carry this important medicinal.

LAVENDER (See description under Essential Oils.)

MARSHMALLOW *(ALTHEA OFFICINALIS)*

Common Names: Common mallow, cheeseflower

Description: The root is where the original "marshmallow" got its name. The spongy root was boiled, sweetened, and eaten as a confection, a far cry from the sugary puff ball in our grocery store today. The plant must be at least two years old before harvesting.

Uses: The simmered root produces a wonderfully soothing mucilage that's rich in calcium and pectin and can be applied to rashy, irritated, dry skin. Combined in a lotion with beeswax and cocoa butter, it makes a moisturizing hand and foot treatment. A bit of the mucilage (made from powdered, dried root and water) combined with essential oil of thyme or tea tree and applied to blisters will help heal raw skin.

Where to obtain: Harvest from the wild if you wish. You may be able to find the dried root from a good herb shop, but definitely through mail order.

MEADOWSWEET *(FILIPENDULA ULMARIA)*

Common Names: Spiraea, queen-of-the-meadow, bridewort

Description: The flower buds contain salicylic acid, which has anti-inflammatory and pain-reducing qualities. Aspirin was originally synthesized from a meadowsweet extract.

Uses: Meadowsweet liniment can be used to help relieve the pain of arthritis. I make mine combined with white willow bark and marshmallow root and use as an external rub for achy joints and feet.

Where to obtain: I usually purchase it powdered to use in liniment making from Jean's Greens (see resources). Also available from better health food stores and herb shops. You can grow it, too; it makes a lovely, fragrant plant.

MYRRH

Common Names: Gum myrrh tree

Description: An aromatic, reddish–brown resin/gum that in ancient times was a common embalming agent and incense.

Uses: Myrrh has antiseptic, astringent, and anti-inflammatory properties. It is used by herbalists today in making liniments to aid in healing open sores, insect bites, and athlete's foot.

Where to obtain: Usually only available through mail order in small resin chunks or powdered form.

PEPPERMINT (See description under Essential Oils.)

PLANTAIN *(PLANTAGO MAJOR)*

Common Names: White-man's foot, broad-leafed plantain, common plantain

Description: A common perennial "weed" that grows nationwide in abandoned lots, roadsides, and lawns. The plant acts as a mild astringent and is slightly mucilaginous.

Uses: The fresh leaves, when crushed, can be applied to sores, abrasions, and bug bites. I like to make an infusion of the dried or fresh leaves combined with comfrey root and blended into a soothing hand and foot cream.

Where to obtain: Harvest from the wild. Just make sure no herbicides have been applied to it and the area is free of dirt and pollution. Also, most herb shops and mail-order catalogs carry the dried leaves.

ROSEMARY (See description under Essential Oils.)

SAGE *(SALVIA OFFICINALIS)*
Common Name: Garden sage
Description: A pretty garden herb with antibacterial and astringent qualities.
Uses: Sage tea makes an excellent astringent wash for acne, oily skin, athlete's foot, and sweaty, odoriferous feet. A deodorizing foot powder can be made from dried, powdered sage mixed with a few drops of essential oil of tea tree, baking soda, and cornstarch.
Where to obtain: Sage is easy to grow and dry. Otherwise, purchase dried sage from health food stores and herb shops, and through mail-order catalogs.

ST.-JOHN'S-WORT *(HYPERICUM PERFORATUM)*
Common Names: Klamath weed, goatweed, hypericum
Description: The top of the plant is covered in a cluster of small, daisylike yellow flowers that have tiny black oil dots on the perimeter of the petals. The small leaves have these dots located sporadically on the surface. These are oil glands that contain the herb's healing properties.
Uses: The fresh flowers make a gorgeous red solar-infused St.-John's-wort oil. You must make some and keep it in your herbal medicine chest. (See the recipe Sweet Relief — Aspirin for the Feet Salve on page 172. This lovely oil with its anti-inflammatory and analgesic properties is used as a base for sore muscle balms and sore foot oil rub formulas. It speeds the healing of bruises, cuts, scrapes, and hemorrhoids.
Caution: The infused oil can cause photosensitivity if used daily for a prolonged period.
Where to obtain: You can try to grow a patch if you wish, but will probably find it easily growing wild in meadows or behind old buildings. The dried flowers are available generally through mail-order catalogs only, but please try to find the fresh flowers; they make the best oil.

THYME (See description under Essential Oils.)

WALNUT, BLACK

Common Name: Black walnut

Description: This deciduous tree grows in the eastern United States. It has rough, dark bark and produces a delicious, oily nut surrounded by a thick rind.

Uses: The bark, leaves, and nut rind produce a very dark brown dye. This liquid can be used as a hair rinse to temporarily darken gray hair and doubles as an antiparasitic astringent to help rid feet and nails of fungus. The powdered walnut rind/hull can be mixed with other powdered herbs and starches to make an antifungal foot powder.

Where to obtain: The fresh product is always preferred, but dried is usually available in better health food stores and herb shops, or through mail-order suppliers.

WILLOW, WHITE *(SALIX ALBA)*

Common Names: Salicin willow, European willow

Description: A graceful tree with flowing, drooping branches whose bark is high in salicylic acid, a relative of aspirin.

Uses: Used by Native Americans in tea form as a pain killer and for bathing to help relieve arthritis pain. An astringent foot bath of chilled white willow tea relieves hot, tired, sore feet, too. I like to make a pain-relieving liniment containing powdered willow stem bark, meadowsweet, and marshmallow root and massage onto stiff joints.

Where to obtain: I have gotten this fresh when my husband has had to remove a dying willow tree from a customer's yard. The dried herb is generally only available through mail-order suppliers.

WITCH HAZEL *(HAMAMELIS VIRGINIANA)*

Common Names: Winterbloom, snapping hazelnut, Virginia witch hazel

Description: Witch hazel produces a woody seed pod that bursts when the flowers are blooming (September through December), making an audible "pop" and casting its two hard black seeds up to 20 feet or so. Now you know where it gets the name "snapping hazelnut."

Uses: A decoction made of leaves, twigs, and bark is highly astringent, light reddish-brown, and great for an oily skin wash, abrasions, insect bites, and poison ivy. It makes a good liniment rub for sore muscles and backs.

A footbath made from a strong decoction of the herb combined with a few drops of essential oils of lavender, tea tree, and peppermint is soothing and refreshing to tired, sweaty feet. It relieves itching, athlete's foot, and helps heal blisters, too.

Where to obtain: Harvest from the woods, but don't damage the tree by removing a large portion of the bark; use a few twigs and leaves instead or order in dried form through mail-order sources.

HOW TO MAKE "REAL" WITCH HAZEL

Since the publication of my first book, *The Herbal Body Book* (Storey Publishing, 1994), I have received many requests for instructions to make "real" witch hazel, which is superior to the store-bought product. The drugstore version contains approximately 14 percent alcohol and the balance is water with only a small percentage of the original witch hazel properties. Here is my recipe:

WITCH HAZEL TINCTURE

  8   tablespoons (120 ml) dried witch hazel leaves, bark, and twigs or
       16 tablespoons (230 ml) fresh, crushed leaves and twigs
  2   cups (460 ml) 80-proof vodka (any brand will do fine)

To make:
1. Place the witch hazel and vodka into a widemouthed jar, tightly cap and store in a dark place to macerate (soak) for 4 weeks
2. Shake daily.
3. Strain and store in decorative bottles or dropper-topped bottles.

To use:
1. To 1/2 cup (120 ml) of water add 2 dropperfuls of tincture. The tincture can also be applied full strength to all skin irritations, even open wounds, but it can be very drying with prolonged use.
2. Wash affected area as necessary.

Storage: There's no need to refrigerate witch hazel, and it will last indefinitely.

Yield: approximately 2 cups of concentrate

WINTERGREEN *(GAULTHERIA PROCUMBENS)*

Common Names: Checkerberry, Canada tea, mountain tea, spiceberry

Description: Wintergreen has analgesic, astringent, and stimulant qualities. The essential oil is produced from the leaves and fruit and contains methyl salicylate, a relative of aspirin.

Uses: Essential oil of wintergreen can be irritating, but if used thoroughly diluted, is a good rubbing compound for muscle aches and tired, sore feet. I like to use the dried, powdered leaves in foot powders, and to make a strong tea for use in footbaths to relieve minor aches and pains, and reduce foot odor.

Where to obtain: Ethically harvest from the wild, picking only what you need. Never deplete an area of the plant when harvesting. Leave plenty of strong plants so there will be lots of herb for you to use at a later date. If unavailable, it is usually only found in better herb shops and through mail-order catalogs.

YARROW *(ACHILLEA MILLEFOLIUM)*

Common Names: Milfoil, soldier's woundwort, herbe militaire, nose bleed

Description: Yarrow is a pretty garden perennial with white, yellow, or pink flower heads and a pungent fragrance. It is frequently grown as an ornamental.

Uses: The leaves are bitter and astringent with antiseptic, anti-inflammatory, and pain-relieving properties. A strong tea makes a wonderful foot wash for hot, sweaty feet and athlete's foot. The leaves, stems, and flowers can be made into an astringent, healing tincture to be applied full strength to cuts, blisters, and open wounds. Yarrow has properties similar to German chamomile, very soothing and healing. It also helps stop bleeding.

Where to obtain: Plant a few flowers of this beautiful and beneficial plant in your perennial bed. The dried herb can be ordered through mail-order catalogs. Better herb shops may carry it also.

THICKENERS

When making herbal creams, lotions, and salves at home, natural thickening agents are necessary to give the product its desired texture, ranging anywhere from a thin, lotionlike consistency to a very thick paste salve.

The following ingredients are commonly used by herbalists and kitchen cosmetologists to soothe and moisturize the skin, as well as to help bind the recipe ingredients together.

BEESWAX

Description: Beeswax comes from the honeycomb. It can range in color from deep golden yellow to creamy white. Most white beeswax is refined and is imported from China. The wax I use comes straight from the apiary. It's deep yellow, unfiltered, speckled with tiny bits of plant debris, and smells strongly of honey. Thus, most of the products I make with it also smell like honey and have a yellow cast, unless I add a strongly scented essential oil that overpowers the honey aroma.

Uses: I use beeswax to thicken and stiffen lotions, salves, lip balms, and creams. It also acts as an emulsifier to help bind oils and water together.

Where to obtain: Mail-order sources are your best bet, though a few herb shops and health food stores carry it. Craft stores usually carry the sheets, but these can be very expensive. Try Champlain Valley Apiaries (see resources). That's where I buy mine and also my honey.

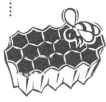

COCOA BUTTER

Common Name: Chocolate tree

Description: Cocoa butter is derived from the tropical cocoa tree. The beans or seeds are pressed to produce cocoa butter. It's solid at room temperature, but melts when applied to the skin. It is also relatively stable, not prone to rancidity.

A bonus characteristic of cocoa butter is that it smells like chocolate! When combined in a basic salve with unfiltered, fresh beeswax, the result is a sensory delight. It smells sweet and rich and chocolaty. You'd think you were rubbing a Hershey bar on your body!

Uses: Cocoa butter acts as a lubricant, skin softener, and emollient. It will not harden a product like beeswax, unless the room temperature is cold, but will thicken and make a rich, creamy, moisturizing product. Cocoa butter is great for dry, cracked skin in winter and used plain as a lip conditioner. I like to use it in overnight foot treatments to help heal severely dry, cracked, thick skin.

Where to obtain: Health food stores and herb shops, better drugstores, and through mail order. Buying in bulk, as with anything, saves you money.

GLYCERINE, VEGETABLE

Description: Glycerine is a by-product of the soap-making process. Available from either animal or vegetable sources, it is an oily, very thick fluid that has a sweet, warm taste.

Uses: Used as a solvent, humectant, and emollient in cosmetics. It absorbs moisture from the air, thus keeping moisture in creams and on your skin. Glycerine can also be used as a cough syrup base.

Where to obtain: Through most health food stores and through mail order. Drugstores carry glycerine, but the bottle doesn't usually designate the source.

LANOLIN, ANHYDROUS (WITHOUT WATER)

Common Names: Wool fat, wool wax

Description: Lanolin is the fatty secretion from the sheep's oil glands taken from the wool after shearing. It is a yellow, semi-solid fat that acts as a natural emulsifier and water–absorbing base. Lanolin holds water to the skin and is easily absorbed.

Uses: A great emollient used in making dry skin creams and lotions, lanolin is good for normal to dry skin. I usually use liquid lanolin, a very thick, viscous, oily liquid, when making natural personal care products.

Where to obtain: Better health food stores, herb shops (occasionally), and definitely through mail-order sources.

SALTS AND STARCHES

The ingredients represented in this section are derived either from plants or minerals. They are primarily used as a base for making herbal foot powders and soothing bath salts.

ARROWROOT

Common Names: Obedience plant, maranta starch

Description: Arrowroot powder is made by grinding the thick plant rhizomes into a starchy, white, fine powder, similar to cornstarch, that is soothing and nutritious.

Uses: I use it as a base for foot and body powders.

Where to obtain: Any grocery store carries arrowroot, but it can be purchased in bulk from some mail-order herb companies.

BAKING SODA

Common Name: Bicarbonate of soda

Description: A white, crystalline, odorless, and salty-tasting alkaline powder.

Uses: Baking soda makes an excellent addition to a footbath for smelly feet, and when poured into stinky sneakers it absorbs moisture and odor. Relieves itchy, rashy skin when used in a full-body bath and also softens the water. I also like to use baking soda in making deodorant foot powders, natural tooth powders, and herbal bath salts.

Where to obtain: Any grocery store. Buy the big boxes and save money!

BORAX

Description: A white, crystalline mineral salt excavated primarily from California. Have you ever used a product called "20 Mule Team" Borax Laundry Booster? That's borax! I realize this doesn't sound like a glamorous personal care product, but look at the label on a jar of bath salts — one of the first ingredients is sodium borate. It's all in the packaging!

Uses: Used in liquid cosmetics as an emulsifier. When making lotions and creams, you are trying to get oil and water to mix and stay mixed. Borax acts as a binder and texturizer and when combined with beeswax, oil, and water makes a stable emulsion. There is no separation if the recipe is made correctly. Borax also acts as a natural preservative, whitener, and mild antiseptic.

Additionally, I use it to make herbal bath salts mixed with baking soda. It's very soothing and freshening to hot, tired feet and itchy skin.

Where to obtain: Almost all grocery stores carry the familiar green box in the laundry section.

CORNSTARCH

Description: Cornstarch is derived from dried corn kernels. It absorbs water and is soothing to the skin, but can cause allergic reactions in some people.

Uses: I use this starch as a base for herbal body and foot powders, same as arrowroot. Cornstarch mixed with finely ground, dried German chamomile flowers and a few drops of essential oil of lavender makes a gentle powder for infants and adults alike.
Where to obtain: Available in all grocery stores.

EPSOM SALTS

Description: Epsom salts gets its name from Epsom, England. It is a white, crystalline magnesium salt.
Uses: Epsom salts can be used in a foot bath for relief of pain from minor sprains and bruises. Add to this a few drops of your chosen essential oil, depending on what you're in the mood for.
Caution: Daily use can be drying to the skin.
Where to obtain: An inexpensive item to purchase, always available in drug stores, pharmacies, and better grocery stores.

SEA SALT, EXTRA FINE

Description: True sea salt comes from the ocean rather than being mined from the ground. The water is evaporated from it. It's said to have more natural trace minerals than standard processed salt from the grocery store. It rarely contains anti-caking agents, sugar, or whiteners.
Uses: I mix it with baking soda and various essential oils to make herbal bath salts. It leaves your skin with a clean, fresh feeling. Sea salt added to foot baths helps relieve itching and helps dry up oozy sores resulting from poison ivy and athlete's foot.
Caution: Daily use can be drying to the skin.
Where to obtain: Health food stores and mail-order suppliers.

MISCELLANEOUS

The following items do not fit into any of the above categories, though they are still very important when it comes to making natural personal care products.

ALL-VEGETABLE SHORTENING

Common Names: Crisco, Spry, generic vegetable shortening
Description: A creamy, semisolid white hydrogenated vegetable fat. Most vegetable shortenings consist of 100 percent soybean oil or a combination of vegetable oils.

Uses: Use vegetable shortening if you need a shortcut in making the standard beeswax, herb water, borax, and oil, cream or lotion formula. Shortening is already spreadable and sinks right into the skin when applied. All you have to do is add the necessary essential oils, stir, and voilà! An instant cream! Great for you men who don't want to fuss and make herb products in the kitchen.

Where to Obtain: Available in all grocery stores.

BENZOIN

Common Name: Gum benjamin

Description: The fragrant, yellow-beige resin (gum) is thought to exude from injuries to the bark of trees of the genus *Styrax*.

Uses: Benzoin is frequently used in tincture form when making cosmetics and employed as a preservative. It can be used as an antiseptic and astringent skin wash for pimples and open sores. It makes a stimulating footbath when the essential oils of camphor and eucalyptus are added. The powdered resin is sometimes used in making foot powders to treat athlete's foot and foot odor.

Caution: The powder, if inhaled, may cause respiratory allergies.

Where to obtain: I've been able to locate the tincture and resin only through mail-order catalogs.

IODINE, TINCTURE OF

Description: Iodine is a bluish-black mineral mined from the earth.

Uses: Used in diluted form, in an alcohol base, as an antiseptic and germicide in cosmetics and on cuts and scrapes.

Where to obtain: Any drugstore or grocery store carries this product.

VINEGAR

Common Name: Apple cider vinegar

Description: Vinegar can be made from many foods, apples being the main one, then grapes and rice. All vinegar contains between 4 and 6 percent acetic acid.

Uses: I use raw, apple cider vinegar in baths to relieve itchy rashes and sunburn and to soften my skin. In the shower, I dilute it 50/50 with water and splash it on my face after cleansing to remove soap residue and restore proper pH to my skin. It also helps dissolve dry skin buildup.

It is good in footbaths to help soften corns and calluses and leaves your feet feeling fresh and clean.

Caution: Vinegar may be irritating to sensitive skin and open sores.

Where to obtain: Better health food stores and some mail-order suppliers.

VITAMIN A OIL

Description: Vitamin A oil is a natural, fat-soluble antioxidant derived from animal and fish livers, deep green leafy plants, and red and yellow fruits and vegetables.

Uses: Use directly from pierced capsule on patches of dry skin and warts to aid in healing.

Where to obtain: Health food stores, better grocery stores, and through mail-order suppliers.

WATER, DISTILLED

Description: This type of water is derived from a process of steam distillation that removes most of the impurities and bacteria.

Uses: Used in the cosmetic industry and sometimes referred to as "pure" water. I prefer to use this type of water when making creams and lotions that I plan to keep for two months or more. Regular tap water can harbor undesirable ingredients that can, on occasion, cause your cream or lotion to mold prematurely.

Where to obtain: Grocery and drugstores.

ZINC OXIDE POWDER

Description: A very fine white mineral powder that's insoluble in water and has astringent and antiseptic properties. Generally nontoxic.

Uses: Zinc oxide powder is used in foot powders to keep feet dry and encourage healing of athlete's foot and open sores. It is sometimes used in baby powders to prevent and heal diaper rash.

Where to obtain: Some pharmacies carry the powder, but I purchase it through mail-order chemical and cosmetic ingredient suppliers.

SUPPLIES: BANDAGING AND
CUSHIONING AGENTS

Feet take a lot of abuse from tight, ill-fitting shoes, excessive exercise, or injuries from going barefoot. Sometimes genetics causes us to be predisposed to certain foot problems that can get worse with age. Occasionally our feet need a little cushioning, support, and tender loving care.

Podiatrists and orthopaedists often recommend to their patients various types of bandaging and cushioning materials to treat minor foot problems at home and help prevent them from developing further. All of the following products are available at finer retail and sporting goods outlets, drugstores or pharmacies, and supermarkets.

ADHESIVE TAPE (POROUS AND NONPOROUS)
Description: A white or beige tape that comes in ½-, 1-, 2-, and 3-inch widths.
Uses: Used to hold bandages on an injured foot or ankle. Frequently used as a secure wrap to support weak ankles, arches, and sore heels. The ½-inch strips can hold a corn pad in place and also cover the portion of your foot that is blister prone. Use the porous tape if the area you are covering needs to breathe (e.g., blisters, cuts, etc.) Note: This tape does not stretch, so it will not always stay in place during activity.

ADHESIVE FELT
Description: Thicker than moleskin with soft felt on one side and adhesive on the other.
Uses: Can be cut into any shape to form custom padding for corns, sore callused areas, blisters, bunions, and metatarsal and heel pain.

CORN PADS
Description: Round or oval felt or moleskin pads. Available with or without adhesive. Can be custom made by cutting your own out of a larger piece of adhesive felt or moleskin.
Uses: These pads put a cushion of protection between your sensitive corn and your shoe, relieving the friction or pressure between the two. The corn will then gradually disappear.

ELASTICIZED ADHESIVE TAPE

Description: The same as regular adhesive tape, but stretches and gives with body movement.

Uses: Good for active people because it stretches with foot movement and will hold any added padding and protective cushioning in place. Also, if you get it wet, it will dry and retain its shape. Elasticized tape won't tend to fall off like regular adhesive tape.

GAUZE

Description: An all-purpose foot treatment material, gauze is basically folded cheesecloth. It is usually sold in sterile, packaged squares. Because it is porous, gauze allows whatever is beneath to breathe.

Uses: To cover blister-prone areas and prevent shoes from rubbing you the wrong way. It is also useful for covering any minor injuries to your foot. Gauze should be held in place with elastic or regular adhesive tape, depending on your needs.

GEL PADS

Description: Gel-filled, plastic pads that come in many shapes and sizes. Some are designed specifically as cushioning devices for the heel or ball of the foot. They are also available as full-length cushioning inserts.

Uses: These provide a soothing layer of comfort cushioning between you and your hard shoes. Not recommended for high heels.

HEEL CUP

Description: Made of plastic or rubber and worn inside the shoe to fit snugly around the bottom and sides of the heel.

Uses: Provides thick cushioning and proper heel support to help alleviate plantar fasciitis (heel pain) and the pain of heel spurs. Absorbs and disperses the shock when your heel strikes the ground.

HEEL PADS

Description: Made of foam rubber or foam rubber covered with plastic to cover the bottom of the heel.

Uses: Used to cushion a sore heel. Can be customized into any shape, such as cutting a hole where a heel spur or bruise is so there is cushioning all around the sore spot and the pressure is relieved on the painful area.

INSOLES

Description: Insoles are generally three-quarter-length or full-length padded shoe inserts. They are available in many versions: foam rubber, gel-filled, terry cloth lined, arch support, athletic support, and odor-destroyers with baking soda.

Uses: There's an insole designed for just about every shoe whether you wear high heels, sneakers, or steel-toed construction boots. They provide added cushioning just where you need it most.

LAMB'S WOOL

Description: Silky, smooth, white lamb's wool. It feels very soft, like kitten fur.

Uses: This product feels like silk against your skin. It's great to use on blisters or corns between your toes or to wrap around a toe if you have a blister or sore callus on top. A piece of lamb's wool can also be taped in place if you have a "hot spot" on your heel that is about to blister.

MOLESKIN

Description: Moleskin is thinner than adhesive felt. Cushioned on one side and adhesive on the other, it comes in rectangular sheets. Did they derive the name from the softness of a mole's pelt? My cats have brought me plenty and believe me, they're the softest little critters I've ever felt!

Uses: Can use the same way as adhesive felt (see above).

TOOLS OF THE FOOT TRADE: EQUIPMENT FOR HERBAL FOOT CARE PRODUCTS

You probably already own all of the kitchen gadgets required to make, use, and store your personalized foot care products, with the exception of a few storage containers. I haven't asked you

> **FOOT FACT**
>
> Heel pain is one of the fastest-growing foot problems in America, mostly brought on by increased sports activities.

to purchase anything exotic or expensive, except for the food processor, which is handy but not an absolute necessity.

I am a real stickler about two things when it comes to being a kitchen cosmetologist. First, everything you use must be sterile. If it's impractical to boil the tool or storage container, then run it through the dishwasher or soak it in very, very hot soapy water for fifteen minutes and give it a good scrub. You don't want to encourage bacterial growth in your products.

Second, never use aluminum or copper pans or bowls when making lotions, salves, creams, liniments, or tinctures. These metals can react with the herb and acid liquids in your recipes and leach the aluminum or copper into the foot care formula you're making. At the very least, they can discolor the end product.

Large Equipment

These kitchen tools can range in price from approximately $20 to $175 or so. The fancier, more heavy duty, or more high tech, the more expensive. Don't buy cheap tools; they'll only wear out quickly and have to be replaced, which means they weren't so cheap after all! Middle-of-the-road quality is fine, unless you love to indulge yourself and always buy top of the line.

BLENDER
I use this for making creams and lotions in 1 cup (230 ml) quantities or more. With smaller quantities I have difficulty extracting the product from the bottom. You can also use it to grind oatmeal, nuts, seeds, and herbs, but a coffee grinder does a much better job.

COFFEE GRINDER
This is one of my most used kitchen gadgets. It is the same as a nut/seed grinder. I grind oatmeal, almonds, and beans into powders for facial, body, and foot scrubs. Larger and harder herb pieces can be ground into much finer pieces, though not always into baby-fine powder. Note: Don't grind your herbs in the same coffee grinder that you grind your coffee beans in, or your coffee will have a "wangy" taste and your herbs will smell and taste of coffee!

FOOD PROCESSOR

This can replace the blender and do some nut grinder chores too. Great for thoroughly mixing up a *large* batch of lotion (2 cups or more), foot scrub, or powder.

POTS AND PANS

Use stainless steel, glass, or enamel only, please. It's best to have a variety of sizes, including a 1-pint (460 ml) saucepan and 1-, 2-, 3 , and 6 quart (1-, 2-, 3-, and 6-liter) pots. I use all sizes for melting oils and beeswax to make lotions, creams, and salves, and for boiling water for herbal foot bath teas, and extracting gelatinous substances from herb roots.

Small Tools

These are basic items that make your life simpler. You probably have many of these items in your kitchen. Creating products at home, especially creams, lotions, and salves, sometimes requires a lot of stirring. When choosing stirring devices, try to get instruments that you're comfortable with and that fit into your hand nicely.

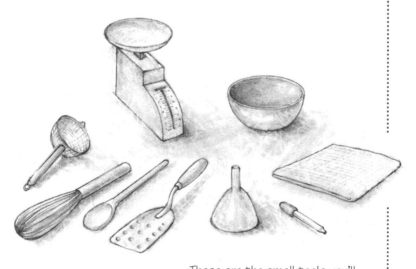

These are the small tools you'll need for making herbal recipes.

BOWLS

From small to large, glass, plastic, enamel, or stainless steel, all come in handy for one recipe or another. I use larger ones for mixing foot scrubs and powders in quantity (usually for gifts) and small ones for single-use or small batches of massage oils, foot scrubs, and foot spray mixtures.

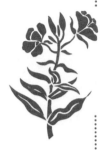

CHEESECLOTH OR HOSIERY

These are for keeping herbal foot bath mixtures from getting in your foot tub. Just place your ingredients into the cheesecloth or hosiery, tie up with string, and let it float about, releasing the beneficial properties while keeping your foot tub tidy. They also make great strainers for herb teas and salves. The hosiery does the best job of screening out fine particulate matter.

EYEDROPPERS

Try to have several glass ones on hand. I use these only as a measuring device for essential oils. Some bottles of essential oils come with their own dropper, but over time the rubber at the end of the dropper will soften and allow air to enter the oils and cause their healing properties to diminish. Always sterilize before use.

FUNNEL

A small funnel comes in handy when pouring herbal recipes into narrow-necked storage bottles. Aluminum foil can be fashioned into a funnel in a snap. No need to worry about the aluminum in this case, because the liquid is in such brief contact with the foil that there's no danger of any metal leaching into the product.

MEASURING CUPS AND SPOONS

You probably have plenty of these standard items for measuring and stirring your herbal concoctions. If not, garage sales and flea markets are good places to buy extras.

SCALE

A tabletop or diet scale is not a necessity, but it's nice to have if you like to know how much your final product weighs. In this book, I don't use ounces as measurements in my recipes, so you can get away without purchasing one. It can be eye-opening to see that 4 ounces (112 g) of German chamomile flowers takes up quite a lot of space versus 4 ounces (112 g) of powdered marshmallow root! It's a nice piece of equipment to have around.

SPATULA

For scraping creams and lotions from blenders and food processors or any type of container, these tools in small and medium sizes are wonderful. I use both narrow and wide blade types. These are also handy for whipping creams, lotions, and salves using the same wrist action you use to beat frosting or egg whites.

STRAINER

When straining herb teas, liniments, and salve mixtures that have large herb matter, I use a mesh strainer. When I need to strain more finely ground herbs, I line it with cheesecloth or pantyhose.

WHISKS

I like to use a large whisk to gently blend large batches of foot and body powder. Whisks mix the herbs and essential oils evenly. Small whisks are super for whipping small quantities of creams, lotions, and salves. I find whisks with a fat handle easier and more comfortable to hold than those with skinny handles.

WOODEN SPOONS

These can be used to stir anything. They are especially good if you're making herbal vinegar–based remedies. The wood won't react with the acid as a metal spoon or whisk might.

Storage Containers

When you make herbal foot care products, you've got to have something to store them in, plain and simple. Choose a container that's aesthetically pleasing and is the appropriate container for the product. See the resource section for herbal mail-order companies that sell storage wares, or look at antique sales and flea markets for old ornamental boxes, bottles, jars, and tins.

BOTTLES

You'll need a variety of these, both plastic and glass, in sizes from 2 to 16 ounces (55 to 454 g). Plastic, narrow-necked bottles with or without a squirt top are the obvious choice for anyone

TOOLS AT A GLANCE

Blender
Bottles
Bowls
Cheesecloth or hosiery
Coffee grinder (nut/seed grinder)
Eyedropper
Food processor
Funnel
Jars
Measuring cups and spoons
Pots and pans
Scale
Shakers
Spatula
Spritzer
Strainer
Tins
Whisks
Wooden spoons

concerned about breakage or someone who travels a lot.

I prefer to use dark cobalt blue, green, or amber glass bottles when I can for two reasons: One, they're pretty (I like the old-fashioned apothecary look); two, the dark-colored glass helps preserve the volatile oils of the herbs and essential oils inside. Make sure the bottles you choose have tight-fitting tops.

JARS

Widemouthed canning jars, ½ pint-, pint-, and quart-sized (230 ml, 460 ml, and 1 l) are perfect for making infused herbal oils, liniments, and tinctures. Use screw-top glass or plastic jars in sizes from 1 to 4 ounces (28 to 112 g) for storing foot scrubs, salves, and creams.

SHAKER JAR

Plastic culinary herb containers from the grocery store can be recycled and used for your powders. The inner top is usually full of holes, perfect for dispensing herb powders. Glass containers are harder to find, but nice to have. Cardboard cylinder shakers are usually sold through herbal mail-order suppliers.

SPRITZER

A must-have for your cooling foot sprays, spritzers are available in 1-, 2-, 4-, and 8-ounce (28-, 55-, 112-, and 228-gram) glass or plastic bottles. Hair spray bottles can be recycled for this purpose.

TINS

Tins have a lovely old-fashioned appeal and look very attractive if decorated with a custom-made label. I like to use these to store dried herbs, foot and body powders with a puff, and dry foot and body scrubs. Tins are available in sizes from ¼ ounce to 8 ounces (7 to 228 g) and larger and sold in better hardware, herb stores, and through mail order.

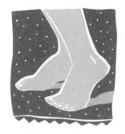

CHAPTER 4

PAMPERED FEET

Professional and at-home foot grooming is a trend that is growing by leaps and bounds. In fact, it's the fastest growing category in personal care today. People are finally realizing that well-cared-for feet are key to a comfortable and healthy body.

According to many salon owners I surveyed, of the nail care services booked by customers, approximately 30 percent are for pedicures. The percentage is increasing every year, especially the number of male customers. Pedicures aren't just for women anymore!

The typical pedicure customer is a woman in her fifties — she's tired, she's raised her kids, and now it's time to splurge on herself. Younger women and those over sixty make up the next largest segment of clientele. Far fewer men feel comfortable in a nail tech's hands. Police officers, an occasional construction worker, and elderly men make up a small percentage of the nail tech's customers. But once they've had a pedicure, so I'm told, they want to come back for more!

A SALON PEDICURE

If you're looking for an hour-long slice of heaven, pay a visit to your local salon and bare your sole to the resident nail technician for a glorious foot-pampering session. I guarantee you'll fall in love with this treatment. If I had extra money each month to spend on anything, I'd have a pedicure. They're simply addicting!

I've given and received scores of facials, back treatments, manicures, lash and brow tints, and makeup lessons, but not until July of 1997 did I partake of a pedicure. I'm a little foot phobic: My feet aren't the most beautiful of creatures so I don't really like anyone deliberately looking at them, except my mother. I rapidly discovered that I'm not the only one who's embarrassed by her feet. Beautiful, perfect feet are rare indeed.

Better salons offer an extensive menu of foot services for tired, neglected paws, ranging from a basic pedicure and optional polish to moisturizing, therapeutic paraffin dips to reflexology (see chapter 8, Foot Reflexology), to acrylic toenails. Yes, you read correctly. If you're not happy with the shape of your natural nails or they've become misshapen as a result of injury, toenails, like fingernails, can be artificially altered. The procedure is a tad expensive, but at what price beauty?

Professional Procedures: Fifteen Steps to Perfectly Pampered Paws

My first pedicure was performed by LeeAnne Sullivan, owner of Cosmetique in Hyannis, Massachusetts. The following is a description of that wonderful treatment. Remember that salons vary in their procedures, and each nail tech follows her own special sequence and adds her own unique personality to the pedicure.

WHAT TO LOOK FOR BEFORE REMOVING YOUR SHOES

◆ Does the nail tech have a current license?
◆ Is she or he clean and well groomed?
◆ Is the salon neat and tidy and does it have a professional setting?
◆ Are tools sanitized and sterile? Ask what cleaning solution the salon uses. Ninety percent isopropyl alcohol is frequently the disinfectant of choice. Each state has its own set of rules and regulations regarding tools and cleanliness. Some require that the salon have a separate set of tools for each customer and others simply require two to three sets of tools: one in current use, and the other two in a sanitizing solution for a minimum of twenty minutes in readiness for the next customer.

Prior to your pedicure, the nail tech will ask you to remove your shoes, socks, or pantyhose and roll up your pant legs. Weather permitting, wear open toe sandals or flip-flops to the salon. Your feet will feel so good when the nail tech is finished that you'll prefer to remain as barefoot as possible. Also, if you have your toenails painted, they're less likely to smear.

As I entered the nail room, I was encouraged to take a seat in one of the thronelike chairs with a built-in whirlpool foot bath and vibrating seat. Not all salons are this fancy, though. Some still use a basic foot tub and chair.

Step 1: My feet were sprayed with 90 percent alcohol disinfecting spray and wiped with a towel. Your nail tech has no idea where your feet have been!

Step 2: My feet were inspected for bunions, cuts, corns, ingrown toenails, and fungus. I was asked if I had high blood pressure, heart problems, or diabetes. If you suffer from any of these conditions you should not be subjected to vibrating chairs or whirling foot baths with alternating hot and cold temperatures or foot massage. Treatments such as these can upset your blood sugar and increase circulation, which *may* prove harmful.

She also inquired as to whether I was a runner, had any circulation problems, or any sensitive areas.

Step 3: My feet soaked in a foot bath for about 5 to 10 minutes to soften and further disinfect them. Tea tree shampoo was used in my vibrating foot bath.

Step 4: My feet were rinsed and dried with a soft towel.

Step 5: At this point old polish is usually removed. I wasn't wearing any.

Step 6: My toenails were perfectly clipped straight across and filed, leaving a bit of the white "free edge" showing.

Step 7: "Calluses grow as a defense mechanism. They're there for a reason," Ms. Sullivan said as she gently shaved off my thickest calluses and pared down the rest with a foot file.

Step 8: Next came an industrious foot and calf massage with a deliciously scented kelp and aloe vera gel sloughing cream to rub the rough stuff off my soles and grind off any extra skin. My feet were then rinsed.

Step 9: My toenails were scrubbed with a small toenail brush to remove any debris and the cuticles were pushed back with an orange stick. Ms. Sullivan recommends using diluted bleach for removing real filth, dirt, and tar from your feet if need be. It's a super disinfectant.

Step 10: More sloughing and massaging followed. Ahhhh!

Step 11: My feet were re-soaked for about five minutes more in a warm whirling tub. I was trying to keep from falling asleep!

Step 12: I then received another fabulous foot and leg massage with peppermint lotion. LeeAnne really used her muscle! The toe pulls were heavenly! I felt like crawling into bed after that! I was completely de-stressed.

Step 13: My legs and feet were next rubbed with cool water and dried. This brings down the temperature of the legs and lowers the circulation a bit. Toenail polish dries faster on cool toes. My feet were also sprayed with 90 percent rubbing alcohol again. You can never be too clean!

Step 14: Ms. Sullivan usually applies polish at this point, but I opted for the natural look instead.

BENEFITS OF A PEDICURE

There are many reasons to visit your local nail tech. She can smooth your calluses and soothe your nerves, cleanse your feet, rev up your circulation, and shape your toenails. Physical touch is of special benefit to the elderly who are often lonely and longing for companionship. Additionally, older individuals often neglect their feet because they aren't limber enough to bend over anymore, aren't strong enough to cut their hard toenails, or simply because their eyesight isn't what it used to be. Overgrown toenails, or club nails, often result from this neglect.

Step 15: Last she fluffed on powder with a large brush to dry, freshen, and fragrance my legs and feet. I felt footloose and fancy free!

HOME PEDICURE

Granted, a home pedicure isn't as luxurious as a professional one, but it is a wonderful way to give yourself a little TLC. It's beautification and relaxation rolled into one treatment.

A pedicure makes your feet look and feel great.

Even if I've had an absolutely awful day at work and am emotionally drained, just knowing that my hands and feet are well manicured and looking spectacular gives me the feeling (even though it's superficial) that I do still have the upper hand, that there is a bit of order in this chaotic life of mine. You might be surprised to find that I'm not the only person to think this way. We are many!

I give myself various foot treatments several times a week. I use a salt and extra-virgin olive oil foot scrub once a week, file my callused areas with a pediwand two to three times per week, trim and/or file my toenails once a week, massage in a thick foot cream twice a week for a night treatment, and use a foot and face mask at the same time once a week to soften and remove dead skin. I have high-maintenance feet and they need the care, but I also *enjoy* "fussing" (as my husband calls it) or "pampering" (as I call it), and taking good care of myself.

PROFESSIONAL TIPS TO KEEP FEET IN SUPER SHAPE

◆ Use a good sloughing lotion two to three times per week to keep dry, flaky skin at bay.
◆ Smooth your calluses with a good foot file or rasp one to two times per week.
◆ Inspect toenails once a week and trim and shape as necessary.
◆ Have a professional pedicure once a month if possible.
◆ Walk, walk, walk, walk . . . .

Consistent and proper care of anything — be it your face, hair, hands, or feet — pays high dividends in the long run. You'll stay more youthful-looking longer and be more comfortable to boot!

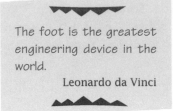

The foot is the greatest engineering device in the world.

Leonardo da Vinci

Equipment Needed

Here's a list of the basic items you'll need to give your feet the royal treatment. I'm sure you have most of them in your bathroom and you can make the others from my recipes.

- ◆ Foot tub. It's a good idea to have two of these, so one can be used as a rinsing bath. They should be big enough so you can swish your feet around a bit. The simplest are large plastic tubs, but you can get fancy and buy a vibrating whirlpool footbath.
- ◆ Towels. Have two of these ready also, one to use underneath the foot tub to catch drips and one for drying your feet.
- ◆ Comfortable chair
- ◆ Toenail clippers
- ◆ Emery board. Use this to file nails and pare down corns.
- ◆ Pediwand, pumice foot rasp, or pumice stone. These three implements do basically the same thing. They give you a real edge when it comes to removing callused and rough skin. The pediwand and rasp are shaped the same, except that the pediwand has coarse sandpaper on one side and fine on the other, and the rasp has an oval pumice stone attached to it. I prefer either of these to a stone because they're much easier to hold.

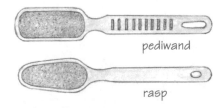

pediwand

rasp

pumice stones

- Orange stick. Used for pushing back cuticles and removing debris under toenails.
- Corn and callus trimmer. This is actually a razor or series of razors with a handle. Used judiciously and with a steady hand, it will remove very thick, hard calluses and the tops of some hard corns. Many men use these when sloughing creams and pediwands just aren't abrasive enough. Be *extremely careful* not to cut too deep and draw blood. Caution: Diabetics should never use this tool.

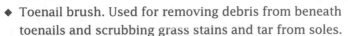

corn and callus trimmer

- Toenail brush. Used for removing debris from beneath toenails and scrubbing grass stains and tar from soles.
- Essential oils. Invigorating oils: camphor, eucalyptus, any mint, tea tree, juniper, bergamot, rosemary, clove, lemon, or orange. Relaxing oils: lavender, geranium, German chamomile, rose, clary sage, almond, or vanilla. You'll need one or more of these to put in your foot bath, foot scrub, cream, and powder.
- Foot powder. Serves to freshen, fragrance, and deodorize feet. Try the Flower Powder recipe on the next page.
- Nail polish, nonacetone polish remover, and cotton balls
- Foot scrub. Try my Autumn Spice Skin Exfoliator recipe on page 67.
- Foot cream. Use this as a massage cream during your pedicure and as a daily softening foot treatment cream. Try making the Lavender Velvet Cream recipe on page 68.

SANITATION OF EQUIPMENT

Your personal pedicure tools should be thoroughly cleansed and scrubbed in hot soapy water, then rinsed with 90 percent isopropyl rubbing alcohol approximately twice a month. If someone in your home has contagious athlete's foot, plantar warts, or toenail fungus, they should have their own set of tools and thoroughly disinfect them as well as their hands and any towels used immediately after performing a pedicure to avoid spreading the disease to other family members. To be on the safe side, the infected family member should store his or her tools in a separate place.

FLOWER POWDER

1/4 cup (60 ml) fine, white cosmetic clay

1/4 cup (60 ml) cornstarch

2 tablespoons (30 ml) finely ground and sifted dried lavender flowers

2 tablespoons (30 ml) finely ground and sifted dried rose petals

2 tablespoons (30 ml) finely ground and sifted dried chamomile flowers

10 drops orange essential oil

10 drops lavender essential oil

10 drops rose or geranium essential oil

Yield: approximately 3/4 cup (180 ml)

To make: Combine all ingredients in a medium-sized bowl.

To use: Sprinkle liberally on feet and legs after pedicure, sprinkle daily in your shoes, or use as a body powder.

Optional: Men can create a more masculine fragrance by omitting the floral herbs and oils and substituting 1 teaspoon (5 ml) cinnamon powder, 1 teaspoon powdered cloves, 1 teaspoon powdered allspice or nutmeg, and 30 drops orange, lemon, or lime essential oil.

Storage: Store in a shaker container or a small box with a puff in a cool, dry place.

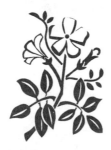

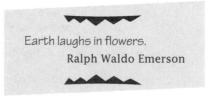

Earth laughs in flowers.
Ralph Waldo Emerson

AUTUMN SPICE SKIN EXFOLIATOR

Here's a fragrant recipe with which to treat your feet. It's great for smoothing out the rough spots on your feet and legs.

½ cup (120 ml) ground oatmeal

2 tablespoons (30 ml) ground almonds or sunflower seeds

1 tablespoon (15 ml) cornmeal

1 tablespoon (15 ml) sea salt

1 tablespoon (15 ml) powdered nutmeg

1 tablespoon (15 ml) powdered allspice

1 tablespoon (15 ml) powdered cloves

1 tablespoon (15 ml) finely ground, dried orange peel

15 drops orange essential oil

10 drops geranium essential oil

5 drops clove essential oil

Yield: approximately 1 cup (230 ml)

To make:
1. Grind the almonds or sunflower seeds and the oatmeal in a nut/seed grinder or coffee grinder until they are the consistency of coarse parmesan cheese.
2. In a small plastic storage container, mix all recipe ingredients thoroughly.

To use:
1. In a small bowl, combine approximately 2 tablespoons (30 ml) of dry mix with 2 tablespoons (30 ml) (more or less) orange juice, milk, rosewater, or plain water until a spreadable paste forms. The amount of liquid you use will depend on how finely ground your herbs and seeds are. Add liquid a little at a time until you get the perfect consistency. The mixture will continue to thicken if you let it stand for a few minutes.
2. Massage onto dry lower legs and feet in circular motions, making sure to get in between toes. Do this for as long as you desire, but at least 5 minutes total, and then rinse. Leaves skin smooth as silk and delightfully scented, too.
Storage: Store dry ingredients for up to one year in tightly sealed plastic storage container away from light and moisture.

LAVENDER VELVET CREAM

This scented cream is a great daily foot treatment. It's one of my favorites.

½ cup (120 ml) all-vegetable shortening

1 teaspoon (5 ml) beeswax

3 tablespoons (45 ml) distilled water, rose water, German chamomile tea, or lavender tea

1 teaspoon (5 ml) borax

15 drops lavender essential oil

15 drops rose or geranium essential oil

5 drops spearmint essential oil (optional, but adds a nice, mild minty note)

Yield: approximately ¾ cup (180 ml)

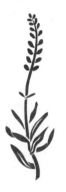

To make:

1. In a small saucepan, heat the shortening and beeswax over very low heat until just melted. Remove saucepan from heat.

2. In another small saucepan, warm the distilled water, rose water, or tea and dissolve the borax in it; then remove saucepan from heat. (To make an herb tea to use as your liquid, simply pour 1 cup [230 ml] boiling water over 1 teaspoon [5 ml] of dried herb, steep 5 to 10 minutes, then strain.)

3. When both mixtures have cooled to approximately the same temperature, set the wax/shortening pan into a bowl of ice cubes and add the essential oils.

4. Drizzle the liquid into it, stirring rapidly with a small whisk or spoon. The cream should set up fairly quickly and look and feel like fluffy cake icing.

To use: Slather it thickly onto clean feet, put on socks, and go to bed. Awaken to "feet of velvet." This product can be used wherever you have dry skin: hands, elbows, knees, or even as a cuticle conditioner. It sinks in amazingly fast, is nongreasy if you don't use too much, and makes your skin super soft.

Storage: Store in an attractive container away from heat or light. No need to refrigerate unless weather is hot. Will last approximately one year if you do choose to chill it or up to three to four months at room temperature.

Do-It-Yourself Pedicure Procedure

Set aside about an hour one evening per week to treat your feet. Surround yourself with all of the necessary supplies so you don't have to keep getting up and dripping water all over the house.

Step 1: A good soak. A footbath is often just as relaxing or stimulating as a full-body bath. The feet are one of the most receptive parts of the body. To your foot tub, add enough hot or cold water or herbal tea of choice to cover your ankles plus a few drops of tea tree essential oil or one tablespoon (15 ml) of bleach to disinfect and a squirt of liquid soap or shower gel. Swish them together. Soak your feet for five to ten minutes to cleanse and soften calluses. Use this time to scrub dirty toenails and soles, too.

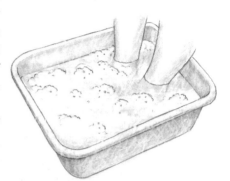

Step 2: After soaking, gently remove calluses with a pedi-wand, rasp, stone, or if you must, very carefully use a callus trimmer. File any corns down with an emery board.

Step 3: Dry feet and legs when finished and remove any old, chipped nail polish now.

Step 4: Try my Autumn Spice Skin Exfoliator (see recipe on page 67) to scrub off any leftover rough skin on your lower legs, ankles, and feet. It feels fantastic and smells great, too!

If you're short on time (and who isn't) whip up the Peppermint Salt Glo exfoliating recipe (see box) instead.

PEPPERMINT SALT GLO

1 tablespoon (15 ml) sea salt
1 tablespoon (15 ml) extra-virgin olive oil
5 drops peppermint essential oil

Yield: 1 treatment
To make: In a small bowl, combine all ingredients, stirring thoroughly.
To use: Massage onto lower legs, ankles, and feet, using a circular motion. Aim for 3 to 5 minutes on each leg and foot. It feels quite invigorating and refreshing and is great to use on a hot summer day!

Step 5: Rinse. Then dry legs and feet with a coarse towel.

Step 6: Coax back cuticles with an orange stick and trim any that are ragged.

Step 7: Trim toenails straight across rather than rounded at the corners so that the white free edge is almost even with the top of the toe. File toenails to smooth any jagged edges.

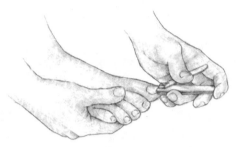

Step 8: Apply foot lotion, oil, or cream and massage in thoroughly for two to three minutes on each foot. Follow the steps in chapter 7, page 104, if you wish.

Step 9: If polishing your toenails, apply a nonacetone remover now to remove all traces of lotion or cream. Now slick on a base coat and two coats of your favorite color, followed by a top coat. There's nothing like ten freshly painted, glossy, perfectly pedicured toes to pick you up and make you feel pretty!

Step 10: After your polish dries, apply your favorite powder to your legs and feet using a large puff or fluff brush to fragrance and prevent perspiration from taking a foothold.

I have two other foot care recipes I'd like to share with you that can be included in your weekly pedicure to add a little variety.

OPTIONAL TOOL FOR DRY LEGS AND FEET

A loofa sponge or coconut fiber brush is wonderful for dry-brushing your legs and feet upon arising each morning and for revving up circulation. If you tend to be plagued with dry skin, a daily brushing starting with your feet and working up to your thighs will quickly banish your scaly skin problem. Remember to wash and dry this tool once a week.

ANTIBACTERIAL FOOT SOAP

1 8-ounce (228-gram)
bottle liquid castile
soap (Available in
health food stores or
from mail-order suppli-
ers. I prefer peppermint
scent, but almond is
nice, too.)
10 drops tea tree essen-
tial oil
10 drops thyme essential
oil

Yield: 8 ounces (228
grams)

To make: Add essential oils to bottle and shake well.

To use: Add a squirt or two to footbath to help clean and disinfect feet and kill bacteria and fungus.

Storage: Will keep in a squirt bottle up to one year.

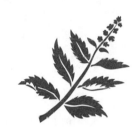

STEP LIVELY SLOUGHING FOOT MASK

The clay in this recipe acts as an astringent, drawing impurities from the feet, and it stimulates circulation and removes dry skin. The apple or grape juice contains natural alpha-hydroxy acids, which also slough and soften skin. It's good for feet suffering from poison ivy, insect bites, eczema, or psoriasis.

3 tablespoons (45 ml)
green clay or bentonite
clay
Enough water, apple, or
grape juice to form a
paste (fresh-pressed
juices are best)

Yield: 1 treatment

To make: Combine ingredients in a small bowl, stirring until a smooth paste is formed.

To use:

1. Apply clay in a medium-thick layer to clean, dry feet, covering them from the soles to the ankles. Allow to dry for 30 minutes.
2. Rinse, then dry with coarse towel.
3. Apply thick cream and cover with socks overnight.

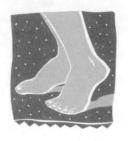

CHAPTER 5

WHAT'S AFOOT?
SELECTING PROPER FOOTWEAR

As a confirmed shoe-a-holic, I was anxiously awaiting the day I could begin doing research for this chapter. I must own nearly forty pairs of shoes, but what type of shoes do you think I wear everyday? My running shoes, my exercise sandals, or my clogs, of course! Why don't I wear my other thirty-seven stylish pairs more often? Because, for extended wearing, they're uncomfortable, they pinch, rub, and generally make my feet hurt.

I work in my home office, so I'm lucky that I can wear whatever shoes strike my fancy or wear none at all, but not everyone is so fortunate. Most people feel that they must succumb to the shoe fad of the moment in order to feel properly dressed for work and that it's an accepted fact of life that your feet must suffer in the name of fashion. Well, in this chapter I hope to educate you as to what foot type you have and what is the best shoe type for your particular foot. There *are* comfortable, fashionable shoes out there that you don't have to be self-conscious about wearing to work.

A BRIEF HISTORY OF SHOES

The first shoes in recorded history were sandals. Nothing fancy, mind you, just purely utilitarian. They were relatively simple to make from abundantly available materials such as straw, wood, or animal hide, and served to protect the wearer's feet from stones, hot sand, and rough terrain.

From the Egyptians to the Greeks to the Native Americans, just about every culture has worn and still wears sandals. They are just as popular and functional today as they were over ten thousand years ago, though a tad more appealing.

Fur-covered and plain leather bootlike foot coverings, as depicted in cave paintings, made their appearance as early as 13,000 B.C., but not until the middle ages did men begin to wear boots as part of their everyday attire. In many "civilized" cultures, women were forbidden to wear functional shoes until the late eighteenth century or so. Until then, they were only allowed to wear dainty slippers or shoes made of fragile materials which were virtually useless outdoors. The one exception was equestrian boots for use when they were allowed to ride horseback.

Early footwear consisted of simple sandals.

I think the worst custom ever inflicted upon women's feet, for the erotic pleasure of their husbands, was the practice of "footbinding." It was an upper-class Chinese custom for hundreds of years to tightly bind the feet of little girls so that they would never grow longer than three inches, in an effort to form a "Golden Lotus" foot. Thankfully, this manner of foot torture was banned in the mid-1900s.

Lotus shoes

Remember the 1970s, the age of Disco Fever and the platform shoe? I loved this style. These shoes made me taller and I found them unbelievably comfortable — after I figured out how to walk in them. They were favored by men and women alike. The pop singer Elton John wore exaggerated versions of this style and must have owned hundreds of wildly colored pairs of stage platforms.

From wedding shoes to prom shoes to bronzed baby shoes to "go-go" boots, shoes evoke memories of the special time they were worn. Styles come and go, but the desire to adorn our feet remains. Shoes are a necessity, a fact of life, but foot torture shouldn't be. There will always be shoe stylists who design the absurd, but many manufacturers are finally coming to the realization that comfort and fashion can be provided in a sensible shoe, which is what I hope you'll decide to wear. Your feet will thank you!

SHOE ANATOMY 101

Ever wonder how a shoe is made? Scores of details (frequently over one hundred operations from beginning to end) go into the development, choice of construction materials, and production of a particular style of shoe, so many that I will only touch on the important basic parts of the shoe that you should be concerned with.

If you think about it, there are really only four categories of shoe styles: athletic, everyday (a broad category), specialized work and safety, and dress shoes. Some of these categories overlap, depending on your field of work and general lifestyle.

In order to select a really good pair of shoes, and to understand what I'm talking about when I mention a certain part of a shoe, you should know a little basic construction terminology, such as where the toe box, heel counter, midsole, upper, medial post, forefoot, shank, and inner and outer soles are.

The style of shoe you choose to wear needs to fit your particular foot anatomy whether wide or narrow, long or short, flat or high-arched. Your foot has to adapt to the shoe environment you decide to put it into, so choose wisely or you will have deformed feet and foot problems down the road.

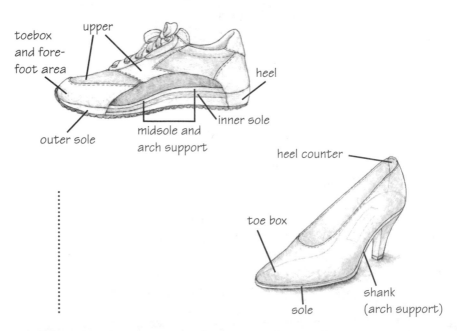

SHOE TYPES

Athletic Shoes
Running
Walking
Cross-trainer
Cleated shoes for track,
    soccer, baseball, or foot-
    ball
Other sports-specific shoes

Everyday Shoes
Basic leather/fabric flats
Leather "dock" shoes
Loafers
Clogs
Sandals
Simple sneakers
Casual boots
Gardening clogs

**Specialized Work and
    Safety Shoes**
Steel-toed construction
    boots and shoes
Cold weather construction
    boots or snow boots
Shoes constructed of non-
    conducting materials
Waterproof, chemical-
    resistant boots and shoes
Dance shoes

Dress Shoes
Men's leather slip-on or lace-
    up shoes
Men's slip-on or zip boots
Women's high-heeled pumps
    and boots

LAST BUT NOT LEAST

A "last" is a plastic or wooden facsimile of the human foot over which a new shoe design is constructed. There is a last created for each and every shoe style and size in existence today. Linda O'Keeffe, author of *Shoes: A Celebration of Pumps, Sandals, Slippers & More,* says that, "After recording as many as 35 measurements from a 'footprint' that shows the distribution of body weight, the [last] maker judges the symmetry of the toes, calibrates the girth of the instep and ball of the foot, and calculates the height of the big toe and the contour of the instep. He also estimates how the foot will move inside the shoe."

Lasts vary from manufacturer to manufacturer. One company's size eight narrow may be another company's size seven-and-a-half medium. As an adult, I've worn as small as a size six-and-a-half medium to as large as a size eight-and-a-half narrow. It's not that my feet are growing and shrinking, it just depends on what style I purchase and who the manufacturer is.

THE LAST WORD

A *board-lasted* or *straight-lasted* shoe gives good motion control. It's the firmest available with maximum medial support and stability aside from a custom-made shoe. It is constructed with an insole board that runs the full length of the shoe. This design helps keep your foot from rolling inward, or pronating, too far and your knees from hurting as a result of excessive pronation. (Some pronation is natural.) How can you tell if the shoes you are buying are made on this type of last? Just turn them over and the sole of the left shoe should look exactly the same as the bottom of the right shoe, without a curve or cutout in the arch area.

A *slip-lasted* or *curve-lasted* shoe has plenty of flexibility throughout the shoe and does not restrict foot motion in any manner. These shoes do not have an insole board, thus providing the greatest possible flexibility and lightest weight. This type of shoe design is good if your foot tends to supinate, or roll outward (also called underpronation). How can you tell if you're buying slip-lasted shoes? Look at the bottoms of both shoes, and it will be easy to determine right from left. There is a definite curve or cutout in the arch area.

A *combi-lasted* or *semicurve-lasted* shoe is a combination of the two types above and is good for an average foot that does not under- or overpronate. It is slip-lasted (cushioned and flexible) in the forefoot and board-lasted (firm and stable) in the rearfoot to control excessive motion.

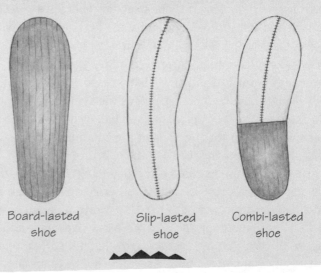

Board-lasted shoe   Slip-lasted shoe   Combi-lasted shoe

I love it when I can buy a so-called "small" size; makes me feel dainty. It's a mental thing, I suppose! The American shoe industry does have standardized sizes, but not every manufacturer adheres to them. That's why it's so important to try on several sizes of the same style before you buy. Don't just ask for a size eight and assume it will fit the same way every time.

It's obvious that a women's dress shoe last would be different from a last for an athletic shoe. The *main* design focus of a dress shoe is the fashion statement it will make. Athletic, specialized work shoes, and flat-soled "comfort" dress shoes are also made with aesthetics in mind, but additionally, they are designed with specific foot types and the activities of the wearer in mind.

If you're one of those people who has difficulty finding shoes that fit properly, despite trying on hundreds of sizes and brands, all hope is not lost. You might benefit from having customized shoes specially made for you, unless you want to suffer from foot fatigue and pain for the rest of your life by continuing to wear mass-produced styles. Consult a podiatrist or orthopedist for professional help and advice.

Women's dress-shoe last

WHAT'S YOUR FOOT TYPE AND THE BEST SHOE FOR IT?

I could fill up an entire book on the technical points of shoe fit, the myriad of high-tech cushioning and upper materials available, and which brand of shoe should be worn for each and every activity that you do in life. But, unless you're a serious athlete, or involved in the shoe industry, a two-hundred-page treatise on every aspect of footwear is not necessary and would need to be updated every few months, besides.

Feet come in all shapes and sizes. Everyone's look a bit different, even in the same family. Foot specialists and shoe manufacturers have decided that these differences can be grouped into three general categories: normal, high-arched, and flat. You will probably fall into one of these or somewhere in between. I'll show you how to figure it all out below.

Buying a pair of shoes shouldn't be a complicated venture. You definitely don't need a medical degree in order to purchase

TWELVE POINTERS FOR PROPER SHOE FIT

These tips, adapted from material from the American Orthopaedic Foot and Ankle Society, will help you buy the right size shoes.

◆ Don't assume you will wear the same size from year to year. The shape of your feet changes with age. Have your feet measured while standing, not sitting, every time you buy shoes.

◆ Buy shoes at the end of your work cycle. Feet tend to swell as the hours go by and will be larger then than right after you arise.

◆ When trying on shoes, be sure to wear hosiery or socks similar to those that will be worn with that pair of shoes.

◆ Try on both shoes, not just one. Most people have one foot that's slightly larger than the other.

◆ If you wear orthotics or any type of special insole, take them with you. These devices take up space intended for your foot so you'll need a roomier shoe than you'd normally wear to allow for proper fit and function of the device.

◆ Walk around on a carpeted surface as much as possible before purchasing. Feet stretch when walking, so the shoes need to allow for movement. Make sure there is adequate space (approximately a finger's width) between your largest toe and the end of each shoe and that the ball of your foot fits comfortably into the widest part of the shoe.

◆ Ideally, the shoe should be shaped like your foot. Make a tracing of your foot and match it to the bottom of the shoe.

◆ The heel should be snug and not slip when you walk. The heel counter should be firm when you squeeze it.

◆ Make sure you can wiggle your toes. They should never feel squished or bound.

◆ The shoe should be reasonably flexible and bend easily at the ball of the foot.

◆ A proper fitting pair of shoes should feel good from the get-go. Don't expect them to stretch. If they're tight when you try them on, then your foot will assume the shape of the shoe and hurt like the dickens!

◆ Make sure they're made of breathable material, such as fabric, leather, or straw. Avoid synthetics without ample ventilation because they trap moisture.

shoes that fit, but a bit of educational advice regarding your specific foot type and what shoes are appropriate for it can go a long way towards ensuring happy and comfortable feet.

In order to match your foot shape to one of the illustrations below, get both feet wet, then make barefoot impressions on a piece of dark wood, medium-colored construction paper, or beach sand. Make sure to stand up straight so that your weight is evenly distributed over each foot. Look at the bottoms of a pair of rubber-soled shoes (preferably) to figure out your shoewear pattern.

The Normal Foot

Characteristics: Normal feet have no extremes. They don't overpronate or supinate (roll too much to the inside or to the outside), and have no arch problems. They're biomechanically efficient. As you walk, your weight falls on the outer side of your heel, rolls a bit onto the outside of your foot, mildly pronates (rolls inward to sag slightly in the arch area), then you push off with the ball of your foot and big toe.

Recommended last: Combi-last or semicurved last.

Recommended shoe type: A shoe with moderate stability and motion control, good arch support, and ample cushioning throughout will suit this foot type just fine. The shoe should not be too rigid or firm nor too flexible and soft.

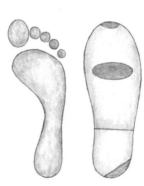

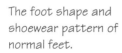

The foot shape and shoewear pattern of normal feet.

The High-Arched Foot

Characteristics: A high-arched foot is often referred to as a supinated or underpronated foot. In this situation, your foot doesn't pronate enough and much of your body weight rolls to the outer side of your foot, putting too much pressure on the bones, tendons, and ligaments in that area, which can result in lower leg and knee problems.

Recommended last: Slip last or curved last.

Recommended shoe type: This foot shape doesn't absorb shock effectively. Shoes with ample cushioning in the forefoot and rearfoot, plenty of flexibility, and minimal stability will encourage foot movement in this more rigid foot.

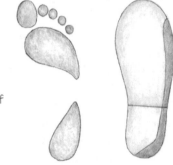

The foot shape and shoewear pattern of high-arched feet.

The Flat Foot

Characteristics: A flat foot, sometimes referred to as a floppy foot, is basically the opposite of a high-arched foot. Instead of your body weight falling toward the outer side of your foot, it rolls excessively inward or pronates excessively, flattening the arch, resulting in a weak foot that can't properly absorb the impact of the body's weight. This can lead to knee, shin, hip, leg, and lower back problems; in fact, your entire body can be pulled out of alignment if you suffer from this foot type.

Recommended last: Board last or straight last.

Recommended shoe type: A motion-controlled shoe with maximum stability, arch support, a stiff medial post (a high-density inner midsole material that extends from the heel to the first metatarsal head, providing pronation control), heel counter (a device that cups the heel and provides rear foot motion and overpronation control), minimal to moderate cushioning, and a wide flared heel will provide the flat-footed individual with the sturdy shoe he needs to help reduce lower body pain and fatigue.

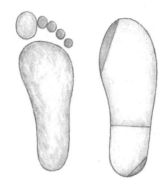

The foot shape and shoewear pattern of flat feet.

Men's Dress Shoes

Men suffer from far fewer shoe-inflicted foot problems than women, primarily because their dress shoes are more sensibly fashioned. They're generally made with a lower heel and wider toe box, with one exception, as I've mentioned before — the stylish leather narrow-toed shoe, which generally has no arch support or cushioning, and squeezes the toes into a pointy "elf" shape.

The best dress shoes for men are top quality wing tips, saddle shoes, dress boots with low heels, and loafers, either slip-on or lace-up. Many shoe manufacturers now make traditional style dress shoes for men, but with an added bonus, walking shoe comfort. These shoes offer foot-cradling comfort and support like a walking shoe, but still look sharp with a suit or nice casual slacks. Several mail-order catalogues offer appealing designs with quality construction (see resources), if you have a hard time finding this type of shoe in your local store.

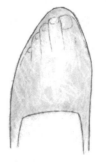
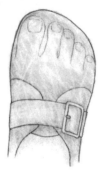

The shoe on the right gives toes more room than the one on the left

Ideally, men should have three pairs of business dress shoes and alternate each day. This minimizes wear and allows the upper and insole to completely dry out between wearings.

Athletic Shoes

Today's athletic shoes are a far cry from the fabric high-tops of the 1950s and they're not just for athletes anymore, either! Sports shoes are one of the top-selling shoe styles made. Modern shoes have gone high-tech and are now designed for every sport and every foot type. If you really need arch support, motion-control, stability, or cushioning, then running or walking shoes are the way to go; they can be purchased according to the particular needs of your feet.

FOOT FACT

It's not necessary to own sports-specific shoes for each sport you play. A cross-trainer will usually do, unless you participate in a particular sport more than three times a week. Then a specialized shoe may be in order (e.g., running, walking, basketball, tennis, aerobic shoes, etc.).

The athletic shoe designer really has one main goal in mind — to produce a shoe that will protect your feet from shock resulting from all that pounding they receive when participating in your favorite sport. This is why you need to be especially careful when purchasing your athletic shoes and make sure to buy a pair made with the last that your foot type needs to help protect your feet from injury.

Safety Shoes

Whatever your career, shoes are an important functional part of your daily "uniform." Physically demanding, high-risk jobs, whether in the construction, agricultural, electrical, sanitation, or chemical field, require special safety shoes to protect your feet from physical harm. In addition, a high quality safety boot or shoe generally gives superior all-around comfortable support for those of you who are on your feet all day.

My husband owns a tree service and landscape construction business, and his steel-toed boots have saved his feet from being crushed many a time. His feet have had everything from boulders to manhole covers fall on them but he's never been injured. Once, one of the stabilizer legs on his backhoe sprang up out of position and practically crushed his foot between it and the body of the backhoe. The steel toe in the boot was crunched a bit, the thick tread, hard rubber sole mangled, and his foot was a bit purple and bruised, but without those fantastically constructed boots, he would have lost his foot and possibly been unemployed for quite some time. Every year he purchases a new pair of his favorite steel-toed boots. They're nearly two hundred dollars, but worth every dollar!

If you work in a potentially dangerous field, ask your employer if they will provide protective shoes. Many employers provide a full uniform, including shoes, but others do not, especially smaller companies. Quality safety shoes don't come cheap, but neither does hospitalization and unemployment resulting from a disfigured foot. Don't try to pinch pennies when purchasing protective shoes. Buy the best pair you can afford. Your lifestyle and your feet could depend on them!

Everyday Casual Shoes

Shoes that fall into this category can range from athletic shoes to sandals to basic flats to loafers. If you get to wear casual shoes to work, consider yourself lucky. Your feet receive minimal abuse, compared to those of other people who feel compelled to wear dress shoes to work. I consider casual shoes to be the most comfortable of shoe styles, provided you stay away from fashionable, pointed-toed varieties.

PUTTING YOUR BEST FOOT FORWARD

Your shoes, friend or foe? That's entirely up to you! The quality and fit of the shoes you choose to wear should have utmost priority when shopping for a new pair. Aesthetic appeal comes next. Unfortunately, almost all of us have our footwear priorities reversed.

Some shoe designs are less abusive than others simply because they allow more foot freedom. I've tried not to mention very many brand names or shoe models in this book unless I felt they were of superior quality and was impressed by the company's standards. Brand names and particular models tend to become dated too quickly. I will make another exception here: Of all the foot specialists I have spoken with and the research materials available to me, the shoe types voted least abusive were flat, open sandals or quality slip-on clogs (such as those made by Birkenstock or Stegmann; see resources on page 177 for address). L. L. Bean and Lands' End (see resources on page 177) also offer terrific sandals and clogs of their own. In these shoe styles, your feet can breathe, toes get a good "gripping" workout, and there's no binding or squeezing. I realize some of you may not care for the aesthetics of these shoes, but they can be most comforting if you suffer from foot maladies and even help correct certain shoe abuse problems, such as hammertoes, corns, bunions, neuromas, metatarsalgia, and sesamoiditis.

Women's Concerns

Nearly 75 percent of a foot specialist's patients are women, and the majority of their problems are shoe-inflicted. This is our own fault, really. We encourage manufacturers to keep producing narrow, pointy flats and heels by continuing to purchase them. Additionally, for vanity's sake, most of us wear shoes that are too small for our feet, in order to have a more "dainty" appearance. Did you know that it's common for a woman of sixty years of age, for instance, to still purchase the same size shoe she wore when she was thirty, even though she knows she should wear a larger size?

SOMETHING TO PONDER . . .

Worn-out shoes or shoes past their prime are often relegated to the realm of gardening and lawn shoes. If you spend even a few hours per week working in your beloved garden or mowing and weed-whacking your lawn, you should wear supportive sneakers or waterproof shoe covers or gardening clogs. Just because you're working outdoors doesn't mean you shouldn't take proper care of your feet.

In the November/December 1997 issue of *Organic Gardening* magazine, *OG* researcher Diana Erney searched for a new gardening clog and found that the Super Birki Clog, manufactured by Birkenstock (see resources), was much to her liking. "It's like you're standing in your bare feet in soft sand," she said. Sounds comfortable, and they come in green!

Whatever shoes you *decide* to purchase for your agricultural activities, just make sure they're super comfortable, flexible, and possibly waterproof, if you happen to work in mucky, wet soil or grass.

Take a gander at the shoes in your closet: Most of them probably offer minimal arch support, stability, or cushioning, except your athletic shoes, and I bet only a few pair fit properly. It's no wonder your feet are tired and achy by the end of the day!

"The most important thing about a shoe is how it makes your feet feel," states a flyer I received from one national brand of women's shoes. It's a simple, yet powerful statement. Unfortunately, though, most of us buy shoes primarily for their aesthetic appeal and we'll put up with a degree of discomfort if it makes our "outfit" look smashing! Over the past decade, though, the tide is changing, thank goodness, due to shoe manufacturers responding to the increasing demand for more comfortable "fashionable" casual and dress shoes.

Heels, it has been said, are a woman's best friend. They give added height and a feeling of power. They elongate the legs and make a woman feel sexier and more appealing. On the downside, high heels also cause our body to become unbalanced. Just look at these illustrations. The body's weight is no longer evenly distributed. It is shifted forward onto the balls of the feet, which dramatically increases the pressure on the toes and arches, instead of on the heels, which were designed to absorb the brunt of the shock. If women were meant to wear heels, wouldn't we have pointed heel bones?

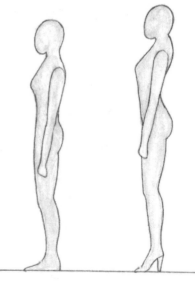

Wearing high heels throws your whole body off balance.

FOOT FACT

The American Orthopaedic Foot & Ankle Society estimates that the effects of wearing poorly designed, poorly fitted shoes costs the U.S. healthcare system (combined with employer costs for employee time lost from work due to foot surgery) as much as $3.5 billion annually!

Because high heels can make you feel glamorous, some people don't want to give them up. Rather than wear heels every day, wear them infrequently, as something special you do for yourself. Wear them on special occasions only, with your best clothes. Just as eating a piece of chocolate cake every day will cause weight gain, wearing high heels every day significantly increases your chances for foot and leg problems. When wearing high heels, limit heel height to two inches or less and wear them only three hours or so at a time, slipping them off occasionally to rest your feet.

Naturalizer and Easy Spirit (see resources) are two common brand names that make shoes on a woman's last, versus a unisex or man's last. A woman's last is generally more contoured and a bit narrower than a man's, affording better shoe comfort. These two companies, in particular, offer athletic and casual shoes with comfort and style in mind, and their dress shoes are designed with a rounder and wider toebox, but still maintain a sleek, fashionable appearance. Also, make sure the shoes you purchase are made of soft, breathable materials such as glove leather, suede, or fabric.

Why settle for a life of discomfort? It's hard enough being a woman these days without having our "dogs" hurt, too!

Children's Shoes

Children's feet grow rapidly and should be measured every time shoes are purchased, from birth through roughly age eighteen, to ensure proper fit. Shoes should be wide enough for toes to wiggle and be made of breathable, natural materials because children's feet tend to perspire profusely.

Infants don't need shoes. Simple warm socks, soft moccasins or booties will suffice. Toddlers, from about nine months to three years, are getting into everything and their chubby legs and wide, pudgy feet aren't the most stable things either. Their shoes should be constructed of soft leather or fabric, have a smooth sole, and be ultra flexible. Lace-up shoes are recommended.

Allow your child to go barefoot as often as possible. This helps to strengthen foot muscles and builds coordination. Children are sometimes a bit awkward in a stiff shoe, especially when playing and running around.

Elementary school children, ages four through twelve, grow like weeds and feel a bit of peer pressure to dress like the other kids so they fit in. Choose styles such as sandals, loafers, saddle shoes, athletic/hiking shoes, or flat-soled dress shoes. It is not advisable to put high-heeled shoes on children in this age bracket. They're too unstable. Just make sure the shoes they choose are well ventilated and don't rub anywhere, since that will cause calluses or blisters.

Teens can find stylish and trendy shoes that fit properly, too. Boys don't usually have a problem finding properly fitting shoes, but girls often want to look "grown-up" and wear pumps and high-heeled clogs. They're not recommended. I wore clogs with three-inch heels during my junior and senior years, and my feet have never looked the same. Sixteen years of age is way too young to start suffering from deformed, cramped, callused toes. Try to steer your child toward heels that are 1½ inches or less. High heels can wait until college.

HOW DO YOU KNOW WHEN TO REPLACE YOUR SHOES?

Shoes that have been worn past their useful life can actually harm your body. If the sole is noticeably worn, then that usually means the midsole, the key shock absorbing part of the shoe, is close to being worn out, too.

Consider this analogy: When the tread on your car's tires begins to wear down, you replace the tires. Worn out tires negatively affect your gas mileage, safety in wet weather, and ability to stop. The same theory can be applied to the "tires" you wear on your feet. Many of you continue to wear your footwear way past the point of replacement. Worn-out shoes have lost their support mechanisms, which can lead to foot, leg, and back fatigue and foot problems. If you exercise frequently or your job demands that you be on your feet all day, it is paramount that you replace your shoes as soon as you notice wear on the outsole. Here's a little tip: Athletic shoes have an approximate life span of about four hundred to five hundred miles of wear and tear. If you run/walk an average of fifteen miles per week, then you should trade those tired shoes in for a new pair about every six to seven months. If you're overweight, they'll wear out even faster.

CHANGING SHOE LACING PATTERNS
CAN PREVENT INJURIES, ALLEVIATE PAIN*

Given all the differences and idiosyncrasies in feet, one lacing pattern for shoes couldn't possibly fit the needs of every athlete. In fact, certain lacing patterns prevent injuries, alleviate pain, and relieve foot problems.

Some General Lacing Tips

◆ Loosen the laces as you slip into the shoes. This prevents unnecessary stress on the eyelets and the backs of the shoes.
◆ Always begin at the bottom and pull the laces one set of eyelets at a time to tighten. This prevents unnecessary stress on the top eyelets and provides for a more comfortable shoe fit.
◆ When buying shoes, remember that those with a large number of eyelets will make it easier to adjust the laces for a custom fit.
◆ The conventional method of lacing, crisscross to the top of the shoe, works best for the majority of athletes.

Seven Lacing Patterns

The following seven lacing patterns alleviate some common foot discomforts.

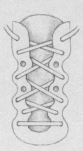

Narrow feet. If you have narrow feet, consider using the eyelets set wider apart on the shoe. This will bring up the sides of the shoe more tightly across the top of the narrow foot.

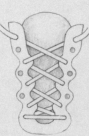

Wide feet. If you have wide feet, consider using the eyelets closer to the tongue of the shoe. Using the eyelets that are closer together will give more width to the lacing area and have the same effect as letting out a corset.

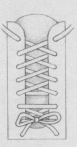

Narrow heel and wide forefoot. If you have a narrow heel and a wide ball of the foot or forefoot, consider using two laces to achieve a combination fit. Use both sets of eyelets to achieve a custom fit that accommodates the width of the forefoot and tightens around the narrow heel. Use the closer-set eyelets to adjust the width of the shoe at the forefoot and the wide-set eyelets to snug up the heel.

Specific pain. If you have a bump on the top of your foot, a high arch, a bone that sticks out, or pain from a nerve or tendon injury, consider leaving a space in the lacing to alleviate pressure. Simply skip the eyelets at the point of pain and draw the laces to the next set of eyelets. This lacing pattern will greatly increase the comfort of the shoe.

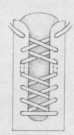

High arches. If you have a high arch, consider lacing your shoes so the laces travel in a straight line from eyelet to eyelet. By avoiding the crisscross method, this lacing pattern creates no pressure points at the laces.

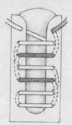

Toe problems. If you have hammertoes, corns, bleeding toes, or toenail problems, consider lacing your shoes so the toe box area is lifted. You can adjust the height of the toe box by pulling on the lace that travels directly from the toe to the top of the shoe.

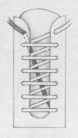

Heel fit. To prevent pistoning of the heel in the shoe and heel blisters, try the lacing pattern shown at right. (Notice the top laces are threaded through each other before tying the shoe.)

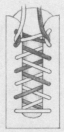

*Carol Frey, M.D., Director of the Orthopaedic Foot and Ankle Center in Manhattan Beach, California, has kindly let me reprint this article on varying shoe lacing patterns. The information is geared toward athletes but can be applied to any type of lace-up shoe.

Socks and Hosiery

Everyone has a preference as to what types of socks or hosiery they like to wear. Socks and hosiery, like shoes, come in a myriad of styles and thicknesses. But, in addition to making your feet and legs look sensational and completing your ensemble, they are designed to wick away moisture and prevent friction between your feet and shoes.

When purchasing socks/hosiery, follow some of the same basic principles of proper shoe fit: They should be well made and loose enough on your feet so that your toes wiggle, but not bunchy so as to cause lumps and creases against your skin. Don't try to save money by buying cheap socks. They're uncomfortable and they don't last nearly as long as a better brand. Try to find seamless brands, which feel better on your feet.

For socks, I prefer natural fibers such as wool or cotton in a medium thickness for year-round comfort. Cotton or wool ragg socks are great for winter wear and thinner varieties for summer wear. If you're athletic or merely walk for your exercise, there are socks made with thicker padding in the heel and metatarsal areas for extra shock absorption and even built-in arch support, too. These feel terrific! Some runners prefer a blend of 70 percent polypropylene, 20 percent wool or cotton, 6 percent spandex, and 4 percent nylon, which is designed to wick away moisture. Many foot specialists recommend the new modern synthetic blends but others still prefer natural fibers. It's up to you and what makes you comfortable.

Men's and women's dress socks are usually a synthetic blend and tend to trap moisture in your shoes. If these socks are not to your liking, try to find a brand that has a greater percentage of natural fibers.

Women's hosiery is generally very thin and made of synthetics. To me, the main function of hosiery is to make your legs look better and help your shoes slip on easier. If you think about it, there aren't really any moisture-absorbing qualities in hosiery. I personally find pantyhose annoying and am

FOOT FACT

The American Podiatric Medical Association states, "In 1994, there were about 140,000 job-related foot injuries, 40,000 of them toe injuries, according to the National Safety Council."

glad I have to wear them only occasionally. Support hose, on the other hand, are a necessary evil for some women with varicose veins and can bring great relief for sufferers of lower leg pain and poor circulation.

Tights can be purchased with a high percentage of natural fiber content. I love to wear these in the colder months under jeans and long skirts.

Orthoses

Orthoses or orthotics are devices that are inserted into your shoe(s) to help correct an abnormal gait or imbalance in your foot. Your foot specialist will usually make a plaster mold of your foot over which to form the orthotic. These devices can be constructed of a variety of materials, such as rigid leather or plastic, semirigid leather and cork, or soft compressible plastic, depending on your needs.

Orthotic devices are also used to treat children's foot deformities. Treatment often begins as soon as the child starts to walk, with the orthotics being replaced as the child's foot grows and foot shape changes.

If you have hard-to-fit feet or have special footwear requirements, your foot specialist may refer you to a pedorthist who works in conjunction with your doctor's recommendations to design and manufacture custom orthotics and/or shoes to ensure that your foot problems are corrected and walking is made a lot more comfortable. If you'd like to receive a listing of board-certified pedorthists in your area, contact the Pedorthic Footwear Association (see the list of helpful organizations, page 180).

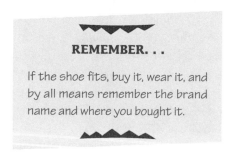

REMEMBER. . .

If the shoe fits, buy it, wear it, and by all means remember the brand name and where you bought it.

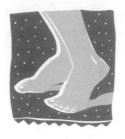

CHAPTER 6

EXERCISES FOR THE FEET

Think back . . . way back. How did you arrive into this world? Were you born with shoes on? Tight socks or hosiery? Did you have corns, calluses, hammertoes, or bunions? No! You arrived buck naked, soft, smooth, and *barefoot*.

In a world void of concrete, asphalt, tar, broken glass, metal, chewing gum, hot pavement, corporate dress codes, or fashion trends, you could continue to go through life barefoot and carefree, or at the very most wear loose sandals in summer and warm, loose moccasins in the winter (some people do). But, alas, most of us do not live in such a place.

For the shoe-wearing masses, specific foot exercises can be of great benefit to strengthen and stretch the muscles of the foot, relieve cramping and strain in the arches, ease heel pain, and the pain of hammertoes, bunions, and toe cramps. Basically, foot exercises can help to counteract the symptoms of footwear abuse.

Some of you may wonder why you need to exercise your feet. You walk a little or a lot during each day, depending on your lifestyle, and that should be sufficient, right? Wrong! This walking that you routinely do is *probably* done in ill-fitting shoes. Even if you wear correct shoes you are still subjecting your feet to some type of rubbing, binding, pressure, or suffocation from lack of air circulation. Your feet, just like the rest of your body, need to be toned and stretched in their natural, unbound state: barefoot. You don't wear your work clothes to run, walk, or go to the gym in do you? You wear something loose and comfortable. So why would you wear shoes when you exercise your feet? Feet should be free and unfettered for at least ten hours per day. If you want your feet to provide you with years of uninterrupted service, treat them with the utmost care. Daily hygiene and a few exercises go a long way toward this goal. Do keep in mind though, that ten to fifteen minutes of foot exercise every day will *not* do any good if you continue to wear ill-fitting shoes that constrict movement and force your feet into unnatural shapes.

THE EXERCISES

The following foot, ankle, and toe exercises can be performed at any time you feel the need to stretch and release tension. If you can't slip off your shoes discreetly during the day, then perform the exercises when you get home from work or finish your daily errands. Slip your body into something more comfortable and slip your feet out of something uncomfortable (your shoes). Relax and unwind. A nice cup of soothing herbal tea, sipped while you do your exercises, tastes especially good, hot or cold!

Footsie Roller Massage

Wooden footsie rollers have been around for many years. They come in all shapes and sizes from single to double or triple rollers. Some are hand held and some sit on the floor. I particularly like the ones with raised ridges going from one end to the other. These are both stimulating and relaxing to my feet. My mother used to use this type when she massaged my feet as a teen. I'd fall asleep on the living room floor before she finished — it felt sooooo good!

If you don't have a footsie roller, a wooden rolling pin can be used in a pinch. Simply place the footsie roller or rolling pin on the floor and while bearing down comfortably, roll the entire length of your foot over the tool, back and forth, and back, concentrating on your arches. Do this for five to ten minutes per foot. This exercise relieves fatigue and cramping, especially in your arches.

FOOT REFRESHER AND DE-STRESSOR

This combined exercise and foot soak is designed to relax tired, aching feet, relieve toe cramps, and strengthen weak foot muscles that support the plantar fascia that runs the length of the bottom of your foot from the heel to the ball of the foot. This one is also good if you suffer from hammertoes and pain in the ball of your foot.

Foot tub
40–60 medium to large marbles
Large towel
2 tablespoons (30 ml) yarrow or sage
2 tablespoons (30 ml) wintergreen
5–10 drops lavender, camphor, peppermint, rosemary, or eucalyptus essential oil
1/2 cup (120 ml) sea salt, baking soda, or Epsom salts

Yield: 1 treatment

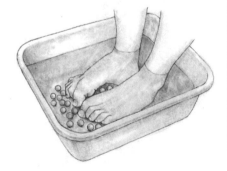

To make:
1. Place the foot tub with the marbles in it in front of a comfortable chair.
2. Boil enough water to fill the foot tub to above ankle height.
3. Remove water from heat and add the yarrow or sage and the wintergreen tightly tied in cheesecloth. Cover and steep for 15 minutes. Remove the herbs. (You can add the spent herbs to your compost pile.)
4. Fill the foot tub with the hot tea, and add the essential oil and the sea salt, baking soda, or Epsom salts. Swish the ingredients around to dissolve the salt and blend in essential oil.

To use:
1. Place your feet in the tub and roll them around on the marbles.
2. Pick up and release marbles with your toes, grasping marbles tightly, squeezing your toes, then releasing. Do this for 10 to 15 minutes.
3. Dry feet roughly with towel.
4. Slather with a thick moisturizer and put on socks.

RELAXING FOOT MASSAGE OIL

After washing and exercising your feet, use this fabulous aromatherapy herbal oil to further enhance your relaxed mode and soften any rough skin as well.

2 teaspoons (10 ml) soybean, jojoba, extra-virgin olive, or almond oil

2–6 drops (depending on strength desired) lavender, German chamomile, orange, or clary sage essential oil

Yield: 1 treatment

To make: Mix all ingredients thoroughly in a small bowl.

To use: Massage into feet using a firm, strong hand. Apply pressure as needed to alleviate fatigue and tension in your feet. Put on socks afterward. You may be ready to climb into bed at this point!

The Golf Ball Roll

This exercise is recommended by Carol Frey, M.D., Director of the Orthopaedic Foot and Ankle Center in Manhattan Beach, California. "Roll a golf ball under the ball of your foot for two minutes. This is great massage for the bottom of the foot and is recommended for people with plantar fasciitis (heel pain), arch strain, or foot cramps."

Point and Flex

This is a great exercise to stretch and strengthen just about everything from your knees down. Sit on the floor, legs stretched out in front of you and palms facing down at your sides. Now point your toes as hard as you can, hold for five seconds, then bend your foot up and curl your toes back as hard as you can and hold for five seconds. Repeat a total of 10 times. If you experience cramping, this usually means that your muscles are weak and need conditioning. Cut back on your repetitions, and gradually work up to 10.

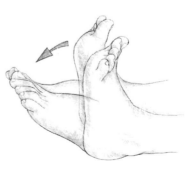

Heel Raises

Heel raises are especially good for women who wear high heels frequently. This shoe type stresses your arches, cramps your toes, and gradually shortens the Achilles tendon, which frequently leads to heel pain when you suddenly switch to a low-heeled shoe and stretch the shortened tendon. Heel raises strengthen your ankle, improve your balance, stretch the Achilles tendon, and provide overall foot conditioning.

This exercise can be performed using a 2-foot-long (60 cm) 6-by-6-inch block of wood or landscape timber or a thick telephone book, or it can be done on the bottom step of a set of stairs or on an exercise bench step. Whatever you use, make sure it's sturdy and won't tip over. Simply hang and lower your heels over the edge of the step, board, or book, as far as comfortably possible to give your heels and calves a good stretch. Now, raise up onto your toes. Go up and down for 20 to 30 repetitions.

An alternate exercise that requires a bit more balance and agility is called standing toe raises. This exercise is recommended by the American Orthopaedic Foot and Ankle Society. Simply "stand on one foot at a time and raise yourself slowly up onto your toes, then lower yourself back down." If your balance is a bit off, hang on to something with one hand to steady yourself. Work up to 20 to 30 repetitions with each foot.

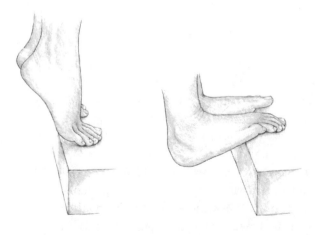

Runner's Stretch

Here's another stretching exercise for high heel wearers that's also good for athletes as a warm–up stretch for their lower leg muscles. It stretches the plantar fascia and Achilles tendon and is good for anyone suffering from heel pain.

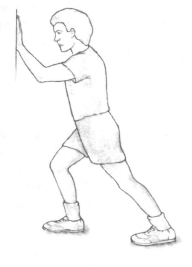

The runner's stretch is somewhat like doing a modified push-up against a wall. Stand approximately 3 feet (.9 m) away from a wall. With your right foot only, take one step about halfway toward the wall. Place palms against the wall at about shoulder height. As you slowly bend the right knee, lean into the wall while keeping both heels flat on the floor. Your left leg should be straight since this is the leg that is receiving the stretch. If you're doing it correctly, you will feel the back of your calf and the arch of your foot stretching. Hold this position for at least 10 seconds. Go back to the starting position, relax, and repeat 10 to 20 times. To exercise the right leg and foot, just reverse positions.

Ankle Strengthener

This particular movement strengthens ankles and helps to relieve stiffness in the ankle joint. It can be performed either by lying on your back and extending your legs up in the air or by sitting in a chair with one leg crossed over the other. I like to do these with a 1-pound (454 g) weight strapped around the middle of my foot. Wrist weights can also be used as long as they are not too tight for your foot. Weights are optional, of course.

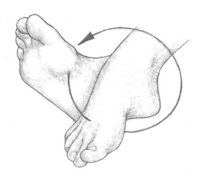

From either position, you simply draw circles with your feet 20 times each first in a clockwise, then counterclockwise, direction. This is a basic exercise, but it feels great at the end of a long day. It is very good as a morning warm-up exercise if you suffer from stiff, arthritic ankles.

Rubberband Big Toe Stretches

This exercise is helpful if you suffer from bunions or toe cramps resulting from wearing shoes with a narrow toe box and/or high heels. This exercise and the following one are also recommended by Carol Frey, M.D., Director of the Orthopaedic Foot and Ankle Center.

Either sit on the floor with your legs stretched out in front of you and your palms on the floor beside or behind you, or sit in a chair with your feet flat on the floor. Place a nice, thick, moderately stiff rubberband around your big toes and pull your feet away from each other. Hold for five to ten seconds, then relax. Repeat 10 to 20 times. If this hurts, or if you have arthritis or bunions in advanced stages, do only as many as you can and gradually increase as your toes gain strength.

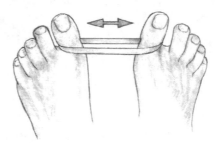

Toe Spreader

You may have seen those little pink foam toe separators used in salons to keep your freshly painted toenails from touching while they're drying. Well, you'll need that little device for this exercise.

Place the separator between your toes and squeeze your toes inward for five to ten seconds, then spread them for five to ten seconds. Relax. Repeat 10 times. This exercise is good for hammertoes, toe cramps, and forefoot pain due to wearing tight, ill-fitting shoes.

Arch Relief

The inner longitudinal arch, which is the arch that absorbs most of the shock of basic daily living, will feel stiff and ache from time to time. This exercise eases the tension and relaxes the muscles in this area.

To perform this exercise, walk on tip toe for thirty seconds, relax, then from a flat-footed stance, roll your feet outward so that you are standing on the outside edges of your feet and remain for fifteen seconds. Repeat 5 times.

Pencil Pick-Up

For those of you suffering from hammer-toes, pain in your forefoot, stiff ankles, or toe cramps, this exercise is for you. It also stretches the tendons on top of your foot. You will need 10 unsharpened pencils and a heavy mug. While sitting or standing, pick up one pencil at a time with your toes and place it into the mug. Repeat with the other foot.

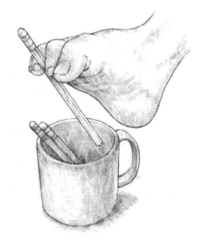

Towel Pick-Up

Both feet will work together for this exercise. It targets the same problems as the Pencil Pick-Up above. Sit in a comfortable chair and place a bath towel on the floor in front of you. Leave it bunched up and somewhat wrinkled so there is some fabric for your toes to grab. Now grip the towel with your toes using both feet, positioned about 1½ to 2 feet (.5 to .6 m) apart. Lift and straighten out your legs in front of you. Hold for ten seconds, then drop the towel. Do 10 repetitions.

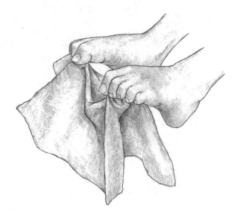

FOOT FACT

Walking is the number one exercise for your feet as well as your body. It strengthens and stretches your muscles, revs up your circulation to help keep your feet warm, and if your feet tend to swell, helps alleviate that problem, too. Barefoot walking is the ideal, but not always possible. So make sure to wear walking or running shoes that are super comfortable and the correct shoe for your foot type (see chapter 5, What's Afoot? Selecting Proper Footwear), then do a few foot exercises when you get home after removing your shoes. Try to get into the habit of walking for health at least four to five times per week and work up to thirty to forty-five minutes each session.

Rocking Horse

This is a multipurpose movement that improves your balance, conditions your entire lower body, and helps strengthen all of the muscles in your feet. You need to be limber and agile for this one or gradually become so.

Stand with feet about one foot apart, with one hand holding onto a chair or bedpost to steady yourself if necessary. Now squat all the way down until you are resting on your tiptoes. Slowly roll back until you are resting flat on your feet, hold for five seconds, then slowly roll forward again until you are on your toes. Work up to 10 repetitions.

I like to do this exercise while doing the "breast stroke" in the air. I squat down on my toes and extend my arms out to the sides for balance. Then as I roll back, I slowly bring my arms forward until they are fully extended in front of me. After I've completed 10 to 20 repetitions, I feel as if I've had a mini workout!

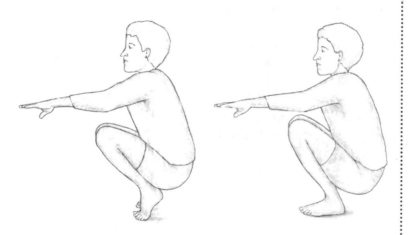

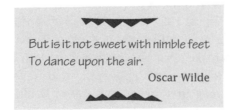

But is it not sweet with nimble feet
To dance upon the air.
Oscar Wilde

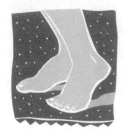

CHAPTER 7

FOOT MASSAGE:
SWEET RELIEF FOR TIRED FEET

If your nerves are frayed, your energy level is running on empty, and your feet have seen better days, then by all means partake of an aromatherapy foot massage. It will soothe your spirits, reduce your stress, put the spring back into your step, and soften your feet. What's good for the body is good for the "sole"!

Take a good look at your feet after they've spent a day in snug leather shoes. What do they look like? Feel like? Do your toes look fresh and happy? Are your feet pink and healthy and rarin' to go and run about? Probably not. More than likely your ten toes are squished against each other, resembling sardines in a can. The skin of your feet looks lifeless, perhaps gray in color and slightly clammy to the touch. I don't think your feet are in the mood to respond positively to, "Tennis anyone?"

"If people bound and gagged the entire body the way they do their feet, none of us would live to the age of twenty," states Gordon Inkeles and Murray Todris, authors of *The Art of Sensual Massage.* If you think about it, they're probably right!

In the August 1997 issue of *Life* magazine, there appeared a wonderful article entitled, "The Magic of Touch: Massage's healing powers make it serious medicine," written by George H. Colt and Anne Hollister. Try to put your hands on a copy if you can. It's eye-opening! In it the authors state, "The idea that touch can heal is an old one. The first written records of massage (the word comes from an Arabic word meaning *stroke*) date back three thousand years to China. A bas-relief on the tomb of Ankh-mahor, an

Egyptian priest who lived around 2200 B.C., depicts a seated man receiving a vigorous foot rub. Hippocrates, the Greek physician known as the father of modern medicine, was a fourth century B.C. proselytizer for massage. "The physician must be experienced in many things, but most assuredly in rubbing," he wrote.

BENEFITS OF FOOT MASSAGE

Regardless of whether you're on the receiving end of a foot massage or you're the one giving it, you both will experience many benefits. Even if you are simply massaging your own feet, it can still be a rewarding and satisfying way to end your day.

TECHNIQUES OF FOOT MASSAGE

A foot massage can be performed at any time you wish or as a part of your home pedicure procedure (see steps in chapter 4, page 69). The following illustrations depict some standard foot massage techniques that a nail technician might perform on her client during a pedicure. If you do not have a willing partner to give you a massage, never fear. These techniques are just as easily done (with a minor bit of alteration) by yourself on your own feet.

If a partner is involved, have the one receiving the foot massage recline against a big pillow on the sofa or bed to fully relax the entire body. Foot massage feels really great if the whole body is at ease.

If you're going solo, find a comfortable chair, preferably one with padded arms and a foot rest, such as a recliner. Sit back, prop one foot in your lap and let the other rest extended in front of you, and massage those feet until they smile or else you fall asleep!

Note: If using massage oil or lotion, a towel or two will come in handy to protect furniture and clothing.

Rub oiled or creamed hands together vigorously to warm them before beginning foot massage. Complete all six steps on one foot before moving on to the other.

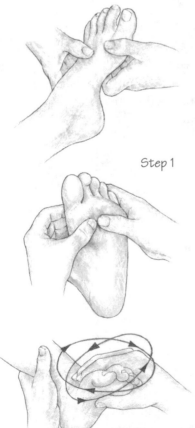

Step 1

Step 2

Step 1: Stroking. Stimulates circulation and warms the foot. Holding your partner's foot in your hands, on the top of the foot begin a long, slow, firm stroking motion with your thumbs, starting at the tips of the toes and sliding back away from you, all the way to the ankle; then retrace your steps back to the toes with a lighter stroke. Repeat this step three to five times.

Now stroke the bottom of the foot with your thumbs, starting at the base of the toes and moving from the ball of the foot, over the arch, to the heel and then back again. Use long, firm strokes, slightly pressing the sole with your thumbs as you stroke. Repeat this step three to five times.

Step 2: Ankle Rotations. Loosens joints and relaxes feet. Cup one hand under the heel, behind the ankle, to brace the foot and leg. Grasp the ball of the foot with the other hand and turn the foot slowly at the ankle for three to five times in each direction. With repeated foot massages, any stiffness will begin to recede. This is a particularly good exercise for those of you suffering from arthritis.

Step 3: Toe Pulls and Squeezes. Toes, like fingers, are quite sensitive to the touch. I find this massage step unbelievably calming. Grasp the foot beneath the arch. With the other hand, beginning with the big toe, hold the toe with your thumb on top and index finger beneath. Starting at the base of the toe, slowly and firmly pull the toe, sliding your fingers to the top and back to the base. Now repeat, but gently squeeze and roll the toe between your thumb and index finger, working your way to the tip and back to the base. Repeat these two movements on the remaining toes.

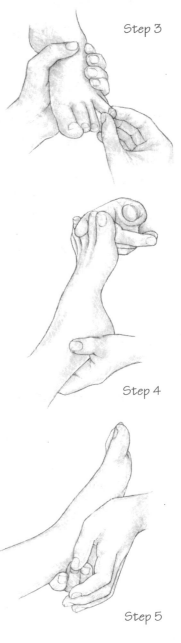

Step 3

Step 4

Step 4: Toe Slides. Grasp foot behind the ankle, cupping under heel. With the index finger of the other hand, insert your finger between toes, back and forth for three to five times.

Step 5: Arch Press. Releases tension in the inner and outer longitudinal arches. Hold foot as you did in step 4. Using heel of your other hand, push hard as you slide along the arch from the ball of the foot toward the heel and back again. Repeat five times. This part of the foot can stand a little extra exertion on your part, just don't apply too much pressure.

Step 6: Stroking. Repeat Step #1 above. This step is a good way to begin and end a foot massage.

Step 5

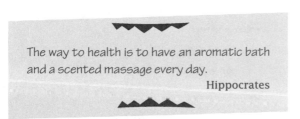

The way to health is to have an aromatic bath and a scented massage every day.

Hippocrates

FOOT MASSAGE ELIXIR RECIPES

Foot massage can be performed with or without oils and creams. It's easier to grip your own or your partner's foot if it's dry, but I prefer to use a small amount of oil or cream fragranced with the essential oils I feel I need at that moment, and massage it in well, because my feet tend to be on the dry side. Don't overdo it, though, or the foot you are working on will be too slippery and difficult to hold.

The following recipes are very easy to make and have a relatively long shelf life in case you decide to double or triple the formula and store it for later use. The ingredients are especially good for dry, neglected feet and will leave your paws exceptionally soft and pampered. Enjoy!

POST-WORKOUT FOOT MASSAGE OIL

This formula will help feet feel cool and refreshed and aid in deodorizing.

2 teaspoons (10 ml) castor, soybean, jojoba, or extra-virgin olive oil
1 drop peppermint essential oil
1 drop eucalyptus essential oil
1 drop rosemary essential oil

Yield: 1 treatment

To make: Combine all ingredients in a small bowl. Stir thoroughly.
To use:
1. Use approximately 1 teaspoon (5 ml) per foot and massage in completely.
2. Put on socks after massage to absorb excess oil and soften feet.

Nothing can cure the soul but the senses, just as nothing can cure the senses but the soul.

Oscar Wilde

SWEET FEET AND CANDY LIPS

This may seem like a strange name for a recipe, but after first making it, I thought it smelled so good, I had to try some on my lips. It's yummy! It's the vegetable glycerine that makes it taste super sweet as well as act as a fabulous foot or lip conditioner.

During a visit to my grandparents over the Thanksgiving holidays, I showed my grandfather this new formula, and he asked if it would help heal the dry, scaly sores on his hands. They'd been there for over six months without responding to any of his doctor's creams. That evening, after wearing my cream for a few hours, he told me that this was the first time his "spots" had remained soft all day. I encouraged him to keep applying the formula as often as possible. He called it "vanishing cream" because it rapidly sank into his skin without a trace of greasiness. I gave my grandmother a pedicure and foot massage using this formula, and the skin on her feet became very soft.

After making this recipe, you may think it's too thick for a massage cream, but because it contains cocoa butter, it will soften and revert to its liquid state on contact with skin.

2–3 tablespoons (30–45 ml) cocoa butter (use the larger amount if you want a stiffer massage cream)

3 tablespoons (45 ml) soybean, almond, jojoba, or extra-virgin olive oil

2 tablespoons (30 ml) vegetable glycerine

20 drops peppermint, spearmint, or orange essential oil

Yield: 4 ounces (112 g)

To make:
1. In a small saucepan, gently melt together the cocoa butter, oil, and vegetable glycerine over low heat.
2. Remove from heat and add essential oil. Stir to blend.
3. Immerse the pan in a cold water or an ice cube bath to make the mixture congeal. Stir vigorously with a whisk. It should become pale yellow and thick quite quickly.
4. Spoon it out into a 4-ounce (112-gram) jar. It will continue to harden, especially in cool weather.
To use: I use about a teaspoon per foot. Scoop out a marble-sized chunk and rub it between your hands to soften and warm, then massage into clean, dry feet.

AGONY OF THE FEET RELAXING MASSAGE OIL

2 teaspoons (10 ml)
  castor, jojoba, soybean,
  or extra-virgin olive oil
3 drops lavender essen-
  tial oil
1 drop German
  chamomile essential oil
1 drop geranium essen-
  tial oil

Yield: 1 treatment

To make: Combine all ingredients in a small bowl. Stir thoroughly.

To use:

1. Use approximately 1 teaspoon (5 ml) per foot and massage in completely. Inhale the aroma on your hands before you massage, and continue to breathe deeply, as these particular oils are extremely calming.

2. Put on socks after massage to absorb excess oil and soften feet.

WHEN NOT TO RECEIVE A FOOT MASSAGE

Since foot massage increases the circulation, it may do more harm than good if you suffer from high blood pressure, a heart condition, or have had a stroke. Most nail technician training courses recommend that people with these conditions consult their physician prior to receiving a foot massage.

CHAPTER 8

FOOT REFLEXOLOGY

I studied reflexology in 1987 and learned The Original Ingham Method as taught by the International Institute of Reflexology (see resources on page 177). This particular method of reflexology was developed by Eunice Ingham Stopfel (1889–1974) in the mid-1930s. Her teachings are carried out today by her nephew Dwight C. Byers.

While taking this course, we were encouraged to memorize Mr. Byers' definition of reflexology. He states, "Reflexology is a science that deals with the principal that there are reflex areas in the feet and hands which correspond to all of the glands, organs, and parts of the body. Reflexology is a unique method of using the thumb and fingers on these reflex areas."

Ponder this: When your feet hurt, what is the first thing you do? Remove your shoes and rub the spots that are sore, right? If you've got a backache, you stretch and try to rub between your shoulder blades or lower back. These are instinctive reflexes on our part to try to increase circulation to the area that's hurting or tense and massage out the pain. Frequently it helps.

Reflexology, though, is not to be confused with massage, which comprises mainly muscle and soft tissue work. Yes, there are many similarities, such as stress relief, increased local circulation in the area being worked on, and similar beginning and ending relaxation techniques, but that's where the similarities end. A reflexologist believes that the entire body can be mapped out on the feet and that the body is

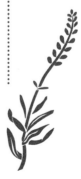

divided into ten longitudinal zones or energy zones that run the length of the body from head to toe, five on each side of the midpoint, and end at the toes and fingertips (see illustrations on pages 111–113). Each zone can be stimulated by applying finger pressure or an acupressure technique to nerve endings and reflexes or trigger points in a corresponding area on the foot or hand. Therefore, if zone one is worked on, then every organ, nerve, ligament, bone, muscle, and tendon that falls into that zone will be stimulated, any energy blockages opened, and vital energy released, reducing stress and creating homeostasis (balance) in that zone. A good practitioner will always perform reflexology on one entire foot, then repeat the procedure on the other foot, and not work on just one zone because most body parts overlap zones.

Exactly why reflexology works is not completely understood, though sound theories abound. We do understand that stress plays a vital role in our health and well-being and that this ancient healing method greatly reduces its effects, thus allowing improved functioning and greater blood flow in the areas suffering from stress-related disease.

HISTORY OF REFLEXOLOGY

Andrea Murray, of the Reflexology Center in Scarborough, Maine (see resources on page 177), is a certified reflexologist and herbalist. In her opinion, reflexology (also known as *zone therapy*) is a "transcultural phenomenon." Many ancient cultures such as the Egyptian, Chinese, Japanese, Babylonian, and others have practiced some type of therapeutic foot/hand pressure therapy as a mode of healing for thousands of years.

Dr. William Fitzgerald, an ear, nose, and throat specialist born in Connecticut in 1872, is commonly known as the founder of zone therapy. Dr. Fitzgerald studied the works of the European physician Dr. H. Bressler, testing Dr. Bressler's theories on his patients and discovering that pressure applied to the fingers in various places would work like a local anesthetic in the arm, shoulder, neck, and face, enabling him to perform minor surgical procedures without chemical anesthetics. In 1917, he and his colleague, Dr. Edwin Bowers, wrote *Zone Therapy,* describing their theory and providing illustrations of the ten zones of the body, but not addressing the reflex zones in the feet. It was later that another physician, Dr. Joseph Shelby Riley, created drawings of the reflex points on the feet. All three of these men further developed the theory of zone therapy.

Dr. Riley's assistant, Eunice Ingham Stopfel, carried their work even further by mapping out the entire body on the feet and discovering how particular points on the feet correspond with the anatomy and the zonal layout of the body. Because of her tireless and successful efforts, she is frequently touted as the founder of modern reflexology.

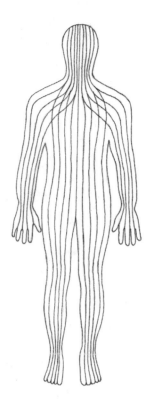

The ten reflex zones of the foot correspond to the ten body zones.

BENEFITS OF REFLEXOLOGY

◆ Promotes relief of stress and tension through relaxation.
◆ Balances the body. As Dwight Byers says, reflexology "helps nature achieve homeostasis." Depending on your individual needs at the beginning of each reflexology session, your body will respond accordingly. For example, if you're sleepy, by the end of the session you will probably feel invigorated; if nervous and tense, then you may feel sleepy and deeply relaxed.
◆ Improves circulation throughout the body.
◆ Enhances nerve function by unblocking nerve impulses.
◆ Helps restore mental alertness by calming the mind.
◆ Helps all body systems to work more harmoniously and to eliminate wastes more efficiently, thus aiding in detoxification.
◆ Bonus: You will never leave a session in a bad mood…guaranteed!

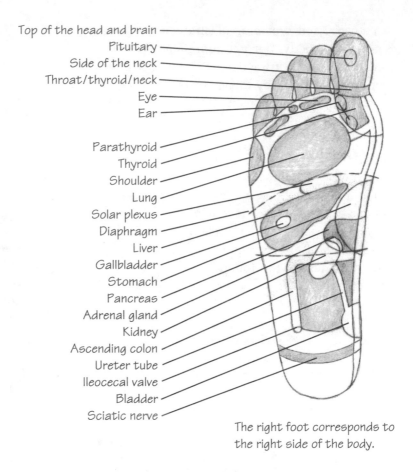

Top of the head and brain
Pituitary
Side of the neck
Throat/thyroid/neck
Eye
Ear

Parathyroid
Thyroid
Shoulder
Lung
Solar plexus
Diaphragm
Liver
Gallbladder
Stomach
Pancreas
Adrenal gland
Kidney
Ascending colon
Ureter tube
Ileocecal valve
Bladder
Sciatic nerve

The right foot corresponds to
the right side of the body.

LET'S UNWIND

"Approximately 75 percent of today's diseases are attributable to stress and tension, [and] various body systems are affected in different ways and to varying degrees. One person may exhibit cardiovascular problems, another gastrointestinal upset, anorexia, palpitations, sweating, headaches . . . to mention but a few of the myriad of bodily reactions to stress. I describe tension as a tourniquet around the body's system . . . a tightening that can lead to serious consequences," says Dwight C. Byers. When tension is released, your muscles cease to contract and the body's systems begin to function more smoothly and efficiently. You feel better all over.

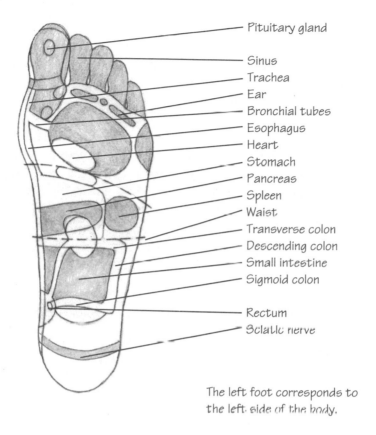

- Pituitary gland
- Sinus
- Trachea
- Ear
- Bronchial tubes
- Esophagus
- Heart
- Stomach
- Pancreas
- Spleen
- Waist
- Transverse colon
- Descending colon
- Small intestine
- Sigmoid colon
- Rectum
- Sciatic nerve

The left foot corresponds to the left side of the body.

Your feet are actually more sensitive and receptive to touch than your hands because they contain a wealth of nerve endings, approximately seventy-two hundred in each foot. Also, because they, unlike your hands, are not constantly exposed to the elements, they are highly responsive to the calming, tranquilizing effects induced by a reflexology session.

I can't show you how to perform all of the various reflexology steps here. You'll need to take a weekend course or study a good book if you're interested in furthering your education (see resources on page 177), but the following are two basic reflexology techniques that can easily be performed at home to bring relief after a stressful day.

All reflexologists have rather short fingernails so as not to inflict stabbing pain to their client's feet. You should at least trim your thumbnails before performing the following techniques.

Big Toe Stimulation

This exercise increases blood flow to your brain, pituitary and pineal glands, and neck. It relieves neck stress and relaxes the mind. Holding your foot in your hand as illustrated, "walk" down and "walk" up each of the five zones in your big toe. In order to "thumb walk" you must use the outside edge of your thumb and bend your thumb at the first joint, then slowly bend and unbend your thumb repeatedly as you climb up or down your toe, simultaneously applying pressure. In other words, cause your thumb to creep along your big toe as if it were an inchworm crawling along your toe. It takes a little bit of practice.

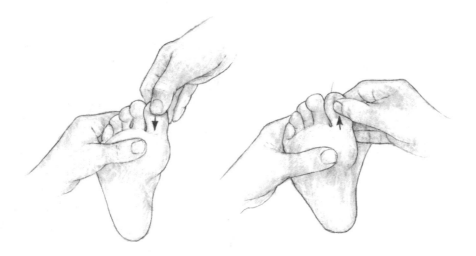

Solar Plexus Press

"The solar plexus is referred to as the 'nerve switchboard' of the body, as it is the main storage area for stress. Applying pressure to this reflex will always bring about a feeling of relaxation," say Inge Dougans and Suzanne Ellis, authors of *The Art of Reflexology*.

To find the solar plexus reflex, grasp the top of your foot and gently squeeze the metatarsals. A depression will have formed just under the ball of your foot and in the center. This depression represents the solar plexus reflex. Look at the foot chart (see page 112) for additional help. Press your thumb into this spot and hold for a few seconds. Release. You may also work your thumb in small circular motions, first clockwise, then counterclockwise. Finish by pressing and holding again.

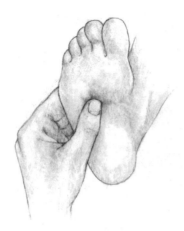

DE-STRESSING FOOT BATH

Begin your mini–reflexology session with a soothing, sensory, and muscle-easing herbal foot bath to cleanse and soften your feet and take the edge off your nerves. I particularly like this one.

Foot tub
German chamomile flowers
Enough water to fill foot
    tub to ankle level
¼ cup (60 ml) Epsom
    salts
¼ cup (60 ml) baking
    soda
1 tablespoon (15 ml)
    borax
3–5 drops lavender,
    German chamomile,
    geranium, or clary sage

Yield: 1 treatment

To make:
1. Use ½ cup (120 ml) of dried German chamomile flowers for each gallon of water. Boil the water, remove from heat, and add German chamomile flowers. Cover and steep 5 to 10 minutes. Strain and cool until comfortable.
2. Pour all ingredients into foot tub and swish with feet to dissolve salts.
To use: Soak feet for at least 10 minutes. Pat dry. Reflexology is best practiced on dry feet.

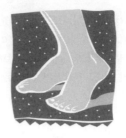

CHAPTER 9

COMMON FOOT PROBLEMS, UNCOMMON REMEDIES

The American Podiatric Medical Association states, "Foot ailments are among the most common of our health problems. Although some can be traced to heredity, many stem from the cumulative impact of a lifetime of abuse and neglect. Studies show that 75 percent of Americans experience foot problems of a greater or lesser degree of seriousness at some time in their lives; nowhere near that many seek medical treatment, apparently because they mistakenly believe that discomfort and pain are normal and expectable."

Happy feet are healthy feet! Locate your foot problem(s) in the following pages and try the recommended natural remedies to help put your feet back on the path to comfort and wellness. If your tootsies need professional care, then follow the suggested foot specialist's advice and visit a podiatrist or orthopaedist if necessary.

To find further foot health information, contact The American Podiatric Medical Association, The American Academy of Podiatric Sports Medicine, or The American Orthopaedic Foot and Ankle Society (see resources on page 177) and ask for their informative foot health brochures. I found them all to be very professional and quite helpful while doing research on this book.

You might also want to look in the Yellow Pages under "Physicians (M.D.)" for an orthopaedic surgeon/orthopaedist, or "Physicians (D.P.M.)" for a podiatrist.

Arthritis

Technically, arthritis is the inflammation of a joint, usually accompanied by pain, an increase in fluid in the joint, and frequently changes in structure and function. It can be a very painful and crippling disease, especially when it manifests itself in the feet. The small joints in your feet are particularly vulnerable due to the load they must carry daily. Approximately forty million Americans are afflicted with arthritis.

Causes and Symptoms: Osteoarthritis, or degenerative arthritis, is the most common form of the disease. It is the result of years of joint stress, injury, and everyday wear and tear. It causes a degeneration of the cartilage in the joints and minor inflammation. Symptoms include stiffness and pain in the joints after heavy exercise, during damp or cold weather, or after you arise in the morning. Osteoarthritis affects one or more joints and is not systemic, unlike rheumatoid arthritis.

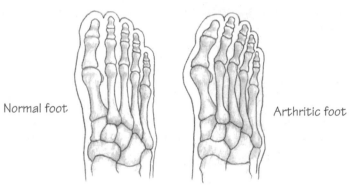

Normal foot   Arthritic foot

Rheumatoid arthritis affects the entire body. It is a chronic inflammatory condition that destroys the cartilage and tissues in and around the joints, sometimes causing the joints to fuse together, resulting in disfigurement and the inability to walk normally. Symptoms can include fatigue, weight loss, extended periods of pain and stiffness, swelling, and redness and/or warmth of the joint. Women are more likely to suffer from rheumatoid arthritis than men.

Rheumatoid arthritis is not completely understood and can be the result of bacterial infection, heredity, suppressed immune system, stress, allergy, or improper nutrition.

Gout is another form of arthritis. It affects men more often than women. It is a condition caused by excess uric acid in the blood resulting from improper protein metabolism, which causes crystals to deposit in the tissues around the joints, forming a very painful, inflamed bump or growth, usually in the big toe.

Treatment: Arthritis is often incurable, but the pain can be somewhat relieved and the progress of the disease slowed with appropriate treatments. For temporary relief, one formula you should try is a product called Deep Tissue Oil formulated by Dr. Richard Schulze, medical herbalist, available from The American Botanical Pharmacy (see resources on page 177). It's a 100-percent-herbal, powerful, deep heating oil that helps relieve pain, inflammation, and stiffness in the joints, tendons, ligaments, and muscles. I think it smells and feels terrific. It makes a great massage oil for the feet. I use approximately 2 teaspoons (10 ml) of my favorite base oil and add one teaspoon of his Deep Tissue Oil to massage my feet and ankles if they feel sore. I don't have arthritis, and hopefully never will, but it sure does make my feet feel super!

Moderate to vigorous exercise (depending on your condition) such as walking, swimming, or bicycling combined with yoga or stretching exercises will help keep joints mobile and your body limber. If you tend to be sedentary, your joints will tend to stiffen with lack of use. It is important to keep as active as possible.

Prevention: Here are some tips to help prevent arthritis from occuring or to at least slow its progression:

- Always purchase proper-fitting footwear. Shoes should be comfortable and supportive, with no binding, pinching, or rubbing that could irritate joints.
- If joints are stiff and inflamed, get necessary rest and stay off your feet until they feel better.
- Try to lose those extra pounds. Extra weight adds stress to weight-bearing joints and can initiate the development of future foot problems.
- Exercise regularly. Stay active and limber.
- Make a habit of having good posture. This keeps your body weight evenly distributed over each foot.
- Keep feet dry and warm.
- Eat a healthful diet.

SOOTHING HERBAL POULTICE

This wonderful herbal recipe helps to relieve the pain and inflammation of swollen joints in the feet. It revs up the circulation and helps ease stiffness and pain. I based it on several formulas I discovered that were used over a century ago. All herbs called for are in dry form.

2 tablespoons (30 ml) plantain leaves
3 tablespoons (45 ml) powdered marshmallow root
1 tablespoon (15 ml) powdered meadow-sweet leaves
1 teaspoon (5 ml) powdered cayenne pepper

Yield: 1 treatment

To make:
1. Combine all ingredients in a medium-sized bowl.
2. Add enough boiling water to form a paste. Stir until you have a gooey consistency and paste feels slippery. Allow to cool a bit if too hot to comfortably touch.

To use:
1. Spread paste on a piece of flannel and place over the swollen joint(s). Wrap the area with plastic wrap. Cover with a warm towel that's right out of the dryer or microwave, if possible. Sit in a comfortable chair, elevate your foot, and relax for about 30 minutes or longer.
2. When finished, rinse your foot and apply a good thick cream to both feet and ankles. Then put on socks.

◆ Avoid a highly stressful lifestyle. Stress can sometimes aggravate an existing arthritic condition.
◆ Avoid smoking, excess caffeine, soda, alcohol, protein, and fat.
◆ Most importantly, keep your doctor informed of any changes in the condition of your feet.

FOOT FACT

According to the American Orthopaedic Foot and Ankle Society, almost half of people in their sixties and seventies have arthritis of the foot and/or ankle.

See a Physician If: If you notice joint stiffness, tenderness, or swelling in your normally healthy feet, visit your foot specialist for a diagnosis. Early diagnosis and treatment may help prevent the situation from developing further.

If your minor arthritis takes a turn for the worse and walking becomes increasingly painful and joints become red or inflamed, by all means schedule an appointment immediately.

Your physician can work with you to design a treatment plan to help preserve joint function or possibly restore it if it's been lost, and help control pain and inflammation. You may want to seek out a holistic foot specialist who uses nutritional and herbal therapies in conjunction with allopathic medicine to help heal your condition.

Athlete's Foot

Athlete's foot is so named because this infection was most commonly seen on the feet of athletes who spent time around swimming pools, steam baths, locker rooms, and showers following exercise. These places are a breeding ground for fungus, and so are your shoes because the environment inside is dark, warm, and moist. Athlete's foot has become more commonplace since the 1970s due to increased interest in fitness and exercise.

Causes: *Tinea pedis*, the Latin name for fungal foot infection, is a skin disease caused by dermatophytes (tiny parasitic fungi) that thrive in warm, moist places. It usually occurs between the toes and on the soles of the feet.

Symptoms: The symptoms can appear rather quickly and can include scaling, flaking, and peeling of the skin between the toes, intense itching, heat, redness, cracking, dryness, and finally the appearance of blisters if the disease is allowed to progress without treatment. The blisters can break and allow the fungus to enter below the skin's surface, thus making the disease even more difficult to treat. Athlete's foot symptoms tend to recur quite easily once you've been infected.

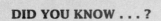

DID YOU KNOW . . . ?

Athlete's foot affects approximately nineteen million adults per year, mostly male.

Treatment: A cure for this miserable skin affliction can sometimes be quite elusive because the pesky fungi can penetrate beneath the skin's surface and be difficult to reach with topical treatments. Because they don't penetrate deeply enough to reach the blood stream, oral medications can have a tough time too. All treatments for athlete's foot should be taken or applied continuously over a period of several weeks to several months until the condition remedies itself.

A simple herbal remedy to try consists of 2 teaspoons (10 ml) tincture of benzoin combined with a few drops of lavender and thyme essential oils, which can help to heal any open cracks on your feet and kill the fungus. Massage this mixture in thoroughly between your toes and on the soles of your feet and allow to dry. Follow this treatment with a good foot cream.

HAPPY FEET

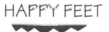

Try this recipe, contributed by an herbalist friend of mine, Jean Argus, to fight foot fungus and odor. It's terrific for active folks!

1 cup (230 ml) cornstarch
2 cups (460 ml) bentonite clay
2 tablespoons (30 ml) powdered goldenseal root
3 tablespoons (45 ml) powdered chaparral leaves
2 tablespoons (30 ml) powdered myrrh gum
4 tablespoons (60 ml) powdered black walnut hulls
3 tablespoons (45 ml) powdered thyme leaves
1 teaspoon (5 ml) peppermint essential oil

To make: Mix all ingredients and add essential oil a few drops at a time, blending well.
To use: Sprinkle this healthful formula daily onto feet and into shoes.
Storage: Store in a shaker container and use within one year for maximum potency.

Yield: approximately 4 cups (1 liter)

Garlic is a potent antifungal and antibiotic and can be used internally and externally in the war against these fungi. Garlic oil can be very effective against athlete's foot and can be purchased in capsule form from the health food store. Simply pierce the capsules and rub the oil onto your affected feet. The oil can also be made fresh at home with this recipe.

ANTIFUNGAL GARLIC OIL

1 cup (230 ml) extra-virgin olive oil
20 peeled and pressed garlic cloves
30 drops tea tree essential oil
15 drops clove essential oil
30 drops lavender essential oil

Yield: approximately 1 cup (230 ml)

To make:
1. Place the olive oil and pressed garlic mash into a small pan over low heat; cover. Allow the garlic to infuse for 1 to 2 hours. The oil should get hot, just shy of a simmer. By then your kitchen will smell pleasantly pungent!
2. Remove from the heat and allow to cool. Strain, add essential oils, and stir. Keep refrigerated in a tightly capped bottle for up to 6 weeks.
To use: You could massage a tablespoon (15 ml) into your feet each morning, put on your socks and go off to work, but the stench would follow you around all day. Instead I recommend applying the oil at night after you've thoroughly washed and dried your feet; then slip on a pair of clean socks and go to bed. I can almost guarantee you won't have any romantic encounters while undergoing this treatment! As the garlic penetrates your feet, it will begin to show up on your breath. This treatment should be performed nightly for approximately 2 to 4 weeks.

Orally, garlic capsules can be taken to boost your immune system and fight the battle from the inside. Allicin, one of garlic's important chemicals, is responsible for its antifungal action. The recommended dosage is four to eight capsules, preferably spread throughout the day, taken with a large quantity of water. Garlic has a tendency to upset sensitive stomachs and cause gas, so you be the judge as to what your tolerance level is. It can't hurt you. The only problem with garlic is that you inherit the lovely fumes along with the benefits.

Prevention: Here are several tips to help you avoid contracting this infection:

◆ Wear shower shoes or rubber thongs when using public showers, walking in locker rooms and around public swimming pools, or lounging around in the steam room. Fungi thrive in these warm, damp, humid places.

◆ Wash and dry your feet daily.

◆ Change socks and shoes during the day if you perspire heavily.

◆ If overweight, lose it. Overweight people tend to sweat profusely, and are more prone to athlete's foot than people of normal weight.

◆ If diabetic, be especially watchful for athlete's foot. The sugar in your perspiration is the perfect feeding ground for fungus to proliferate.

◆ Athlete's foot is contagious to other people as well as to other body parts of your own. To avoid spreading this fungus among us, either dry your feet with paper towels and throw them away or immediately launder your foot-only drying towel in hot water. Bath mats should not be kept in the bathroom if you share this room with other family members. Use clean towels as temporary bath mats and also launder them immediately.

◆ Wear open-toed shoes as often as possible. Feet can breathe and stay drier this way.

◆ Sprinkle a little powder in your shoes daily to keep your feet fresh and dry.

See a Physician If: Several other skin problems can masquerade themselves as athlete's foot, such as a skin allergy or problems resulting from diabetes, circulatory disorders, drug abuse, stress, or poor nutrition. If these have been ruled out and self-treatment is not curing the disease, see a foot specialist or dermatologist immediately. They can prescribe topical or oral antifungal drugs to use in conjunction with all of the above treatments and preventative measures. As with any drug, especially antifungal drugs, there are side effects, which include liver toxicity.

Black Toenails

Causes: Black toenails (subungual hematoma) are caused by an injury to the toenail. Stubbing the toe against a hard object or dropping something heavy on it can cause a black toenail to form. Athletes, especially runners, frequently experience this malady. This toenail injury can occur if their shoes are too short or by running downhill, thus forcing the toes to repeatedly jam up against the inside of the shoe.

Symptoms: As blood pools under the injured nail (this is what causes the black color) and pressure builds, this sometimes results in pain. Most times, black toenails are not painful, just unsightly.

Treatment: Foot specialists recommend a procedure that you can perform at home to release the pooled blood and relieve the pressure under the toenail. Just thinking about this treatment leaves me feeling a bit woozy, but I will mention it here.

The toenail can usually be saved if the blood is drained. First, clean your foot thoroughly, dry, and swab the affected toe with alcohol. Next, heat the end of a needle or a paper clip with a match until it is red hot. If you're brave, now gently pierce your toenail. The heat from the sharp object melts the nail and allows the blood to flow out from beneath it. Follow this procedure with a hot foot bath and add a few drops of lavender or tea tree essential oil as a disinfectant. Dry your feet and swab the toe with alcohol or tincture of benzoin and a drop of tea tree essential oil. If your toenail *does* begin to loosen over time, cushion the nail with gauze and tape it down with an adhesive bandage (don't stick tape to the toenail itself or you may rip the nail off when you remove the bandage). This prevents your toenail from catching on your hosiery or socks.

Caution: Never perform this type of self-treatment if you have circulatory problems or are diabetic. See your physician immediately.

Prevention: The best way to prevent a black toenail is to be more graceful and not drop things on your toes or run into things . . . and also to buy proper fitting shoes. Your shoes should have a roomy toe box that allows your toes to wiggle and has about a half inch of space between your toes and the end of the shoe.

See a Physician If: If you can't possibly envision yourself piercing your toenail with a hot object, or if swelling and infection set in, then see a doctor.

Blisters

Causes: Everyone has had a blister at one time or another. They are caused by friction against the skin from a shoe, abrasive socks, or hosiery and can develop on any part of the foot, even the tips of your toes. New leather shoes are notorious for causing blisters because they tend to be snug until the leather stretches a bit, but any type of footwear can cause a blister, whether the shoe is too big, too short, or too narrow. Runners, walkers, and rollerbladers tend to get more blisters than sedentary folk. All that foot movement and pounding can cause the feet to swell and sweat inside the shoe, resulting in lots of blister-causing friction.

SEASONAL FOOT LESION?

Walter J. Pedowitz, M.D., has found that in his practice, the incidence of black toenails increases dramatically around Thanksgiving and Easter! These are the two holidays when people remove 12- to 18-pound (5- to 8-kilogram) frozen turkeys from the freezer, and drop them square on their big toe! OUCH!

Symptoms: You can actually feel when a blister is beginning to form. The spot gets warm, then irritated, then downright painful if you don't remove your shoe. These whitish pockets of skin filled with clear fluid form between the skin's inner and outer layers in response to friction and can make walking unbearable.

Treatment: There seem to be different schools of thought on whether to pop a blister or not. Some say to leave it alone, whether large or small. Wash the area and swab it with alcohol or iodine; then cover it with an adhesive bandage or moleskin, remove the source of friction, and let nature take her course. Other physicians and sports injury specialists suggest that by popping the blister, especially a large one, healing will take place faster. If a blister breaks on its own, treat the same as if you'd just popped it (see below).

To open a blister, first wash and dry your foot thoroughly. Swab the blister with alcohol or other disinfectant and carefully puncture the edge with a flame-sterilized needle or razor blade. Now drain the fluid, but don't peel off any skin. Allow the layers of skin to adhere. Cleanse with disinfectant again and dry. Apply a bandage, but remove it at night to allow the blister to breathe and dry out, and reapply in the morning after your shower. If it stays moist, healing is postponed and infection can set in.

Caution: Don't attempt self-treatment if you have circulatory problems or are diabetic.

Prevention: Irritating blisters are easy to prevent. Here are some tips for avoiding them:

- ◆ Buy well-fitting shoes. Ideally they should not rub anywhere, even from the beginning. Add insoles or heel cushions if necessary.
- ◆ If you are blister prone or performing lots of physical activity, always wear good socks and apply adhesive felt or moleskin to areas on your feet that frequently blister.
- ◆ Sprinkle powder into shoes and/or socks daily to reduce friction.
- ◆ Some people swear by petroleum jelly or vegetable shortening as a blister preventative. Try the Blister Resister Cream recipe on page 127.

See a Physician If: Blisters are rarely serious. If the blister develops inflammation or an infection, see your doctor immediately.

BLISTER RESISTER CREAM

⅓ cup (80 ml) all-vegetable shortening

10 drops eucalyptus essential oil

10 drops camphor essential oil

Optional: If you're a peppermint lover, like me, you can substitute 15 to 20 drops of peppermint essential oil instead of the above-listed oils.

Yield: about ⅓ cup (80 ml)

To make: Beat ingredients together with a spoon or small whisk.

To use: Apply to blister-prone areas, then cover with thick socks. Helps reduce friction between the sensitive spot and your shoe.

Storage: Store in a small glass or plastic jar and label. Keep refrigerated if not used within thirty days.

BLISTER BUSTIN' FOOT POWDER

This herbal foot powder is simple to make.

½ cup (120 ml) white clay

½ cup (120 ml) cornstarch

1 tablespoon (15 ml) finely powdered sage leaves

1 tablespoon (15 ml) finely powdered peppermint leaves

½ teaspoon (2 ml) clove or peppermint essential oil

Yield: slightly more than 1 cup (230 ml)

To make:

1. In a medium-sized bowl whisk together the clay, cornstarch, sage and peppermint. You can also use a food processor set on the lowest setting if you wish.

2. Add the essential oil a few drops at a time and thoroughly blend.

To use: Sprinkle this spicy powder into your shoes each morning or into your socks to help keep friction, moisture, and odor to a minimum.

Storage: Store in a shaker container and use within one year.

Bunion of the Big Toe

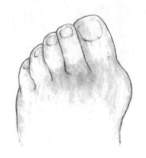

Causes: There is no single cause of a bunion. It may develop from arthritic joint destruction, overpronation of the foot (see chapter 5, What's Afoot? Selecting Proper Footwear), heredity, or from wearing ill-fitting, tight shoes.

Symptoms: A bunion (or hallux valgus) is an inflammation and thickening of the bursa of the joint of the big toe, frequently associated with enlargement of the joint and deformity of the toe. It results in ugly, misshapen feet with the big toe angling in and either tucking under or over your second toe. It is usually painless but can be quite painful if allowed to progress. A bunion has the tendency to increase in size due to excessive weight load and from shoe pressure. It causes widening of the forefoot and may cause your gait to become off-balance. Though not as commonplace, a bunion on your small toe is called a tailor's bunion.

Treatment: Sometimes merely changing the type of shoes you wear can prevent the worsening of a bunion. Whether you are a man or woman, switching from a tight, pointed toe shoe to a sandal can help tremendously. So can wearing a *bunion shoe,* available from most orthopedic shoe stores. Both shoe styles remove the source of pressure on the bunion and have a wider forefront to accommodate a bunioned foot. If you refuse to change shoe styles due to vanity, then your bunion will progressively get bigger, uglier, and eventually painful.

If athletic, you can make a slit in the shoe in the bunion area to allow for extra room and less pressure. If you overpronate, try a commercial arch support to help take some of the weight off the bunion.

Try placing a pad over the bunion to reduce friction. You don't want to add thickness though, as this would just add more pressure, so cut a hole in the middle of the pad where the bunion protrudes. The surrounding area is now built up a bit and hopefully some pressure is taken off the bunion.

Prevention: If bunions run in your family, you can dramatically slow the progression by wearing well-fitting, non-binding, low-heeled shoes with a wide toebox. In fact, everyone should heed this advice. Most of today's fashionable shoes are designed for an elf's foot — long and pointy — not a human's foot. Shoe designers should be ashamed for trying to force your foot into a shape it was never meant to be in and for trying to dictate fashion styles. You should be allowed the freedom to wear comfortable shoes with your work clothes without inciting derision from co-workers and a reprimand from the personnel director.

See a Physician If: If you've tried self-treatment and your bunion is still getting worse and possibly painful, see your foot specialist. He or she may want to rule out osteoarthritis, rheumatoid arthritis, gout, or infection first, as these can also cause pain and inflammation in the big toe. Foot surgery may be required if your bunion is disabling and your foot severely disfigured.

Calluses

Causes: Calluses can be caused from wearing shoes that are too tight, too short, or even too big and sloppy. They can even be caused from going barefoot a lot. Anything that causes rubbing, pressure, or pinching of the skin on your foot can result in a callus. Approximately 14 percent of adults get calluses annually; it's a very common malady.

Symptoms: Calluses are thickened, raised layers of hard, tough, yellow-reddish brown dead skin, oval or elongated in shape, that form on the bottom of your foot, heel, side of your big toe, or even the tips of your toes as a defense mechanism against repeated friction and pressure from rubbing against your shoes or seams in your socks. They can become painful if allowed to grow very thick.

Treatment: The only way to permanently remove a callus is to remove the cause. So unless you're totally sedentary and bedridden, you will more than likely have a callus or two or three on your feet. Calluses return and return, no matter how often you scrape them off. They keep pedicurists in business.

Personally, I use a foot file with medium grit sand paper on one side and fine grit on the other to file down the dead skin on my heels and balls of my feet three times a week. I do this while standing in the shower after the skin has softened a bit. This procedure could also be performed while sitting on the edge of the tub after soaking your feet for a few minutes in ankle-high water. If you add a cup (230 ml) of baking soda or vinegar to the tub, your feet will be even softer. I then dry my feet with a rough toweling and follow with thick moisturizer. I'm very callus prone and this practice keeps my tootsies relatively soft and pain free. A pumice stone can be used in place of the foot file, though I find my file much easier to handle.

Better drug stores carry a tool called a corn and callus trimmer, which is specially made for removing thick calluses. It holds a razor blade or a series of small blades and is used by gently scraping the blade(s) over the softened, callused skin. Extreme caution should be taken when using this tool so that you do not cut too deeply and draw blood.

Moleskin and adhesive felt can be custom cut and placed around the callus to help take the pressure off and relieve the pain and irritation.

Caution: Diabetics, people with circulatory problems, and those with unsteady hands should never attempt to cut or scrape their calluses.

An herbalist friend of mine, Julie Bailey, owner of Mountain Rose Herbs (see resources on page 177), kindly let me borrow her enchanting, mystical recipe for making calendula oil. Try to make 4 to 5 cups (1 to 1.25 liters) of this super healing oil so you can have plenty for other formulas throughout this book. She also sells this wonderful oil ready-made if you're short on time!

"Three days before the moon is full, gather the golden flowers (calendula) after the dew dries but before the noonday sun. Thank the energies, spirits or devas; whom or whichever calls to you. Spread the golden flowers on a screen in a dry, shady and well-ventilated place to wilt and lose most of their water. (They should be leathery not crisp.)

"On the evening of the full moon, select a thoroughly clean glass jar that will be two thirds full with the golden flowers. Choose the best cold-pressed, extra-virgin olive oil. Pour the oil over the flowers to almost three thirds. Put the lid on tight. Dance and sing to the oil. Shake the oil.

"Place your oil in a sun box (greenhouse, hot water closet, black sand pit, etc.). Visit your oil every few days. Dance, sing, and shake. One day before the next full moon, bring your oil into the kitchen. Strain your oil. Bottle every drop into clean dark glass bottles and label.

"Congratulations! You have created and participated in medicine and magic."

This is actually my preferred method of making my herbal oils. It may not be scientific, but I feel that by allowing the universal energy systems to create my healing potion according to their timetable, not mine, I receive a supercharged medicine, a true gift from Mother Earth herself! She provides the medicinal plants and the solar energy. I simply join them together and reap the benefits!

Note: Some water from the herb may still be left in the oil. If, after 2 weeks, you see what looks like dirt in the bottom of the jar of strained oil, that is water settling. This can make your oil go rancid, so pour the oil into a fresh jar, stopping before the "dirt" pours in. You may have to repeat this process a few times until the oil stays clear.

Prevention: There are really only four simple rules to follow to help prevent calluses from forming:

FOOT FACT

People who go barefoot most or all of the time develop thick calluses on the soles of their feet. This is a natural, healthy condition that protects their feet from sharp objects. Less than three percent of aboriginal people (most of whom go barefoot) ever have foot problems, unless from insect bites or injury.

- ◆ Take good care of your feet. Inspect them daily for developing calluses and other foot problems, and treat accordingly.
- ◆ Wear shoes that fit.
- ◆ Don't walk barefoot on hard surfaces such as asphalt or concrete for any length of time or protective calluses will form on the soles of your feet.
- ◆ If overweight, lose it. The combination of excess weight and ill-fitting shoes puts way too much pressure on your poor feet and encourages callus formation.

See a Physician If: If your calluses are not responding to home treatment and keep worsening and become painful, see a foot specialist. Diabetic and elderly people frequently need assistance with foot care because of circulatory problems or because they just can't bend over to scrub the rough spots. Also, the callus(es) may not be just the result of friction, but could be forming because of a foot misalignment problem, which would need to be treated.

CALENDULA BLOSSOM OIL

An alternate, quicker method for making herbal oils is to use the stove method. Here's what you need:

4–5 cups (1 to 1.25 liters) calendula blossoms (wilted in well-ventilated shade for 24 hours)
Extra-virgin olive oil

Yield: About 4 cups (1 liter)

To make:

1. Put the calendula blossoms in a 3-quart (3 liter) pot and pour in enough olive oil to cover by 2 inches (5 cm). The mixture should look almost like a flower-head paste, but with enough oil to allow the flowers to move about slightly.

2. Turn the burner on low. Heat the mixture just below a simmer, and allow to steep for 5 to 10 hours. Don't put a lid on the pot. This only traps in any moisture left in the flowers and will introduce it into your herbal oil, which will encourage spoilage. Check on it every hour or so to make sure the oil isn't simmering.

3. Remove from the heat after the oil smells herby and has attained a rich, golden-orange color.

4. Cool, strain, bottle, label, and refrigerate.

To use: You now have a potent healing oil that can be used as a base in any recipe calling for oil in this book. Try some in the next recipe.

Storage: Will keep 6 months to 1 year if refrigerated. Use within 60 days if not refrigerated.

CALLUS SMOOTHER SCRUB

1 tablespoon (15 ml) sea salt

1 tablespoon (15 ml) calendula oil

5 drops orange or spearmint essential oil

Yield: 1 treatment

To make: In a small bowl combine all ingredients until the salt is completely covered by the oil.

To use:

1. First, soak and wash your feet in order to soften the dead, callused skin. Pat dry.

2. While sitting on the edge of the tub or over a towel or foot tub, massage the mixture into your feet, scrubbing with a moderately firm hand over your callused areas. Do this for as long as you want, but at least 2 to 3 minutes per foot.

3. Rinse with warm water and roughly rub your feet dry. You should now have a moisturizing calendula oil residue remaining on your feet that will penetrate and continue to soften for hours to come.

4. Massage a bit of castor oil into each foot and put on a pair of socks if you want to really pamper your feet.

How beautiful are the feet of those who bring good news!

Romans 10:15

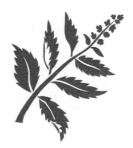

Children's Foot Problems

Many adult foot ailments begin in childhood. This is why it is paramount that you see to it that your child's feet are properly cared for. Neglecting foot health when young can lead to leg and back problems later in life. Children's feet grow very rapidly. By 12 to 16 months, their feet have reached almost half adult size. This is a critical time to really pay attention to foot health and head off any potential development problems.

Children can suffer from some of the same foot problems as adults, including athlete's foot, profuse perspiration and odor, sports injuries, and wounds or scrapes from running around barefoot.

Causes, Symptoms, and Treatment: The causes, symptoms, and treatment of most foot problems are the same in children as adults. However, because the bones in children's feet are not completely hardened, sports injuries can be especially damaging. Their feet are soft and pliable, and excess pressure from playing the same sport over and over or from training too long and hard can cause long-term problems. Your child could become injury prone. Many doctors recommend that the intense, specialized sports training be postponed until the late teens, after growth plates are closed.

If perspiration and odor are a problem, make sure to have your child wash his or her feet two to three times a day, wear clean cotton or wool socks, and sprinkle powder into shoes and socks every day.

FOOT FACT

Have you ever looked at a newborn's feet? They're small and pudgy and relatively flat. All toddlers under 16 months have flat feet. Their arches don't fully develop until they reach seven or eight years of age.

Prevention: Most importantly, make sure your children take a daily bath and thoroughly clean their feet. Check for tenderness, minor irritations, calluses or corns developing (which could be a sign that they are outgrowing their shoes), or rashes (a possible sign of poison ivy or athlete's foot). Trim long toenails. Check to see how their shoes fit. Is there enough room in the toe box for their toes to wiggle? If not, invest in a new pair. And, give them a gentle foot

FUNGUS AMONG US OIL

Here's a nighttime herbal treatment to help clear up athlete's foot in children.

2 teaspoons (10 ml) castor, jojoba, soybean, or extra-virgin olive oil

2 drops tea tree essential oil

1 drop lavender essential oil

1 drop clove or thyme essential oil

Yield: 1 treatment

To make: Stir oils together in a small bowl.

To use:

1. Thoroughly massage the oil into your child's clean feet (the child can do it if older). Concentrate between toes and around cuticles. If only one foot is infected, treat the other one anyway as a preventative.

2. Put on socks and send the little one off to bed. Do this nightly for several weeks until healing takes place.

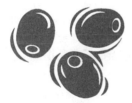

massage once a week if they're receptive. It'll let you take a good look at the condition of their feet, and it's good bonding time to boot!

See a Physician If: If you notice something that looks abnormal in your child's feet, see a foot specialist. Poor posture, an awkward or stumbling gait, toes that turn in or out, knock knees, or bowleggedness can be a sign that something is amiss. Many times a child will outgrow these problems, but it's better to be safe than sorry. Serious deformities such as clubfoot or skew foot should be treated as soon as possible.

DR. MOM'S HERBAL HEALING CREAM

For minor scrapes, scratches, bug bites, and small puncture wounds from running through the woods and stepping on thorns and pinecones, keep this healing cream on hand. It's extremely soothing and moisturizing for your child's playtime injuries as well as excellent for your dry hands, elbows, knees, legs, and feet. It's also the best cuticle conditioner I've ever made!

½ cup (120 ml) distilled water

2 teaspoons (10 ml) chopped comfrey root

2 teaspoons (10 ml) plantain leaves

¾ teaspoon (3 ml) borax

½ cup (120 ml) vegetable shortening

1 teaspoon (5 ml) beeswax

15 drops lavender or geranium essential oil

5 drops orange essential oil

Yield: approximately ¾ cup (180 ml)

Note: If using fresh herbs, decrease the water by 2 tablespoons and double the herb portions.

To make:

1. Add water and herbs to a small saucepan, cover, and simmer on a very low setting for 30 minutes.

2. Add the borax and stir until dissolved. Remove from heat and cool until just warm.

3. While the herbs are cooling, melt the vegetable shortening and beeswax in another small saucepan over low heat until just melted. Do not allow to simmer.

4. Remove from heat and stir in essential oils.

5. Strain the herbs through a mesh strainer lined with pantyhose or cheesecloth, reserving the greenish herbal liquid in a cup. Gently lift the liner material and twist and squeeze the healing, slippery mucilage out into the container. You should have approximately ¼ to ⅓ cup (60 to 80 ml) of herbal formula. Dispose of the herbs into your garden or atop a house plant.

6. By now the herbal liquid and melted vegetable shortening should be approximately the same temperature. While briskly stirring the shortening with one hand, slowly drizzle in the herbal liquid with the other. Continue stirring until creamy and almost firm. If you set your small saucepan over a bowl of ice while performing this procedure, it will set up quite quickly. You should now have an approximate ¾ cup (180 ml) of multipurpose cream. It will have a pale greenish-brown color and smell pleasantly herby.

To use: Apply this cream generously over cleaned, irritated skin. Use as often as you wish. My skin drinks it right up. It doesn't tend to be greasy, unless too much is used.

Storage: Store in decorative glass or plastic jars and refrigerate. Discard if not used within 45 days.

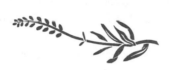

Cold Feet

It seems that women tend to suffer more from cold feet than men. Is it because women frequently wear tight shoes that restrict circulation to the feet? It may be that women in their menstruating years can suffer from iron deficiency, which results in a lower level of oxygen-carrying red blood cells traveling throughout the muscle tissue, impairing circulation to the feet. Whatever the cause, having cold feet can be downright uncomfortable. I've elicited agonizing screams from my husband when I've placed my winter-frigid feet on his toasty back in bed. He hates it, but it feels so good to me!

Causes: Cold feet can also be a result of pneumonia, heart failure, diabetes, malnutrition, injury, or nervous system impairment.

Symptoms: I don't have to tell you how cold feet feel . . . COLD! They are also chilly to the touch, sometimes tingly and a bit numb, and can even be a bit bluish or purple in color due to poor circulation.

Treatment: Walk, walk, walk! Keep those feet moving and your heart pumping as often and for as many miles as possible. The more you move, the better your circulation. That's the key to having warm feet.

Make sure you include plenty of foods containing vitamins A, B complex, C, D, E, and iron, in your daily diet. These nutrients, in particular, strengthen the veins and capillaries and help keep your blood oxygen-rich.

Another remedy that you may have heard of is to sprinkle powdered cayenne pepper into your shoes and socks. This is a stimulating, warming herb and will cause increased circulation to the feet. Mix about 2 teaspoons (10 ml) white cosmetic clay, cornstarch, or arrowroot with 1 teaspoon (5 ml) powdered cayenne pepper and sprinkle away. Be sure to wash your hands thoroughly after handling cayenne. Also, acquire a taste for hot sauce or hot peppers such as jalapeño or habañero. By simply adding these tasty foods to your diet, you will automatically rev up your circulation and add lots of vitamins C and A as well.

Prevention: Here are a few tips to ensure nice warm tootsies:

- Always wear comfortable shoes, never too tight or too short.
- Keep feet warm and dry by wearing socks that breathe; natural fibers are best.
- Get plenty of exercise and fresh air and breathe deeply.
- Eat a nutritious, well-balanced diet.
- If you sit or stand in one position all day long, get up and stretch your feet and legs periodically to keep the blood from stagnating in your legs.

See a Physician If: If you suddenly start suffering from cold feet or are a chronic sufferer and none of the above suggestions seem to help, schedule a doctor's visit. Your doctor may want to rule out a circulatory disorder, anemia, or diabetes.

HOT AND COLD FOOT BATH THERAPY

Here's an invigorating, old-fashioned remedy for cold feet. It wakes up the entire body, too!

2 foot bath tubs
2 tablespoons (30 ml) peppermint leaves
2 tablespoons (30 ml) rosemary leaves
2 bath towels

Yield: 1 treatment

To make:
1. Bring to boil enough water to fill one foot tub. Remove from heat and add herbs tightly tied in cheesecloth. Cover and steep for 15 minutes. Remove the herb bags.
2. Find a comfortable chair and place a bath towel on the floor in front of it and put the foot tubs, side-by-side, on the towel. Fill one tub with the hot herbal liquid and the other with almost icy water. Throw in a few ice cubes if you wish, since you're going to be sitting here for a while.

To use:
1. Put feet in the hot tub first for 3 to 5 minutes (careful, don't scald yourself), then immerse in the cold water for 30 seconds or so. Alternate 2 to 3 times.
2. When finished, briskly rub feet dry with a coarse towel for about 1 minute per foot.
3. Slather on a rich moisturizer, and put on thick wool or cotton socks. Your feet should feel great.

Caution: If diabetic, please don't partake of this foot bath. Because of the temperature extremes, it can potentially cause a sugar imbalance and possible dizziness.

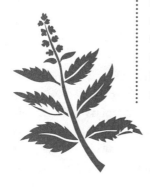

Corns

Causes: If you could go barefoot every day of your life, you wouldn't get corns. Corns are caused by pressure or friction from ill-fitting shoes. But unless you live wild and free in a temperate climate, shoes are a required and necessary part of your dress code. Unlike a wart, a corn does not contain blood vessels or nerve endings. People with a cavus foot type or extremely high arch are often susceptible to this affliction because their toes are pulled back a bit and corns tend to form on the tips and tops of the toes as well.

Symptoms: A hard corn, or *heloma durum,* is a tough, cone-shaped thickening of the horny layer of the epidermis that usually occurs over a toe joint, having a hard, brownish-gray "eye" in the center and surrounded by inflamed skin.

A soft corn, or *heloma molle,* forms between the toes as a result of friction. It is soft because the sweat between your toes softens the normally hard corn tissue. Beneath every corn there is a prominence of the bone, so when your toes are squeezed together, such as when wearing narrow, tight flat shoes or pointed-toe, high-heeled shoes, the bones will rub against each other, causing pressure and irritation. As a result, layers of tissue grow over the pressure point(s) until a corn or two are formed. The constant friction between your toes causes the skin of the soft corn to die or become inflamed, which can lead to very painful walking.

FOOT FACT

Your feet tend to widen and change shape as you age. They should be measured whenever new shoes are purchased to help avoid the development of blisters, bunions, corns, calluses, and other foot problems that can stem from shoes that are too tight or ill-fitting.

Treatment: You can either change your shoe style and take the pressure off your corns so they'll go away on their own, or continue to perform constant maintenance on your existing and new corns.

Corn pads are available from the drugstore. These have a hole cut out of the middle so the padding fits around the corn and the pressure is relieved. Corn pads take up space, so make sure to wear roomier shoes while wearing the pad. Custom pads can also be made from moleskin and adhesive felt, as thick or as thin as you wish, but always put the padding around the corn, not on top of it.

For women who feel they must wear high heels, some pressure can be relieved by placing a metatarsal pad in front of the heads of your metatarsals to prevent your toes from sliding down and jamming into the pointed-toe portion of your shoe. This will reduce *some* of the friction, but definitely not all of it.

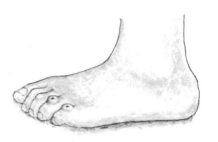

Hard corns form at shoe pressure points.

Some foot specialists disagree as to whether to apply salicylic ointment or drops (also known as corn drops), available from the drugstore, to your corns. The drops *can* help remove the corn, but if any of the acid runs off onto the surrounding skin, it can burn and even cause a hole or ulcer to form. The drops can be applied in the center of the corn pad, but please use with care. **Caution:** Diabetics should never use salicylic acid drops to treat their corns. Ulceration of the skin could lead to serious problems.

In his book *American Folk Medicine* (Meyerbooks, Glenwood, Illinois, 1973), Clarence Meyer includes a corn remedy used by Dr. R. L. Louis in 1877: "Take bark of the common willow, burn to ashes, mix them with strong vinegar and apply to the parts. This is a very effectual remedy for corns or warts." The reason this might work is that acetic acid, the main constituent of vinegar, applied daily to the corn will soften the dead skin and cause the corn to slowly peel away. Straight vinegar can also be used. Try it and see if it works for you.

Other old-fashioned remedies include applying wintergreen essential oil to soft corns and wrapping soft linen around the toe or swabbing hard corns with castor oil and also wrapping with linen. Do these daily until the corns disappear.

Prevention: Stop wearing shoes that pinch or bind. Wear open-toed sandals or comfortable shoes with a wide toe box. Go barefoot as much as possible, either on the grass or beach or around the house, so your feet can expand and relax.

FOOT FACT

Every year approximately 150 million people get corns, though only a fraction seek professional treatment.

See a Physician If: If a corn reaches the painful stage and nothing seems to be helping, your foot specialist can extract it for you. Your doctor can also trim it, if you feel you can't do it yourself, though it is almost certain to return if you continue to wear the same shoe style. If the problem persists, your doctor may need to perform surgery.

Diabetic Foot Concerns

Causes and Symptoms: Diabetes is relatively unknown in poorer countries where food is scarce and overeating is not a problem, but in the United States, the land of plenty, it is one of the major degenerative diseases, afflicting approximately sixteen million people. It is a metabolic disease characterized by high blood sugar and the inability to properly process dietary carbohydrates, resulting in an abnormal amount of sugar in the urine. Health problems, such as cardiovascular disease, obesity, retinopathy, blindness, kidney damage, and circulatory disorders of the limbs and feet, often develop as the illness progresses.

Diabetics frequently suffer from foot problems such as athlete's foot, neuropathy, numbness, cold feet, ulceration, calluses, and corns. It is therefore wise to visit a foot specialist at least twice a year to prevent any minor problems from developing into potentially limb-threatening complications.

Diabetics, like everyone else, can have a problem with athlete's foot, but because the perspiration of the diabetic person is "sweet" from the increased sugar in the blood, it makes a doubly fun place for the fungus to frolic. See "Athlete's Foot" on page 120 for treatment suggestions.

Neuropathy is the gradual loss of nerve function in the legs and feet leading to loss of feeling or sensation. It can also affect the ankles and hands. If you have this disease, you won't be able to feel if you've injured your foot or if blisters have formed from snug shoes. Loss of feeling in the feet of a diabetic can lead to serious problems down the road.

Poor circulation of the lower limbs can slow the healing process. What might start as a minor cut, bruise, blister, corn, or callus could develop into an open sore, infection, ulceration, and eventually gangrene if not properly cared for. Diabetics frequently suffer from cold feet and hands. Your situation

VANILLA FOOT BUTTER

4 tablespoons (60 ml) almond, olive, jojoba, soybean, or calendula oil

1 vanilla bean, chopped into ¼ inch (.6 cm) pieces (available in grocery or health food stores)

1 tablespoon (15 ml) beeswax

2 tablespoons (30 ml) cocoa butter

1 tablespoon (15 ml) anhydrous lanolin

20 drops geranium, rosemary, or peppermint essential oil

Yield: approximately ½ cup (120 ml)

To make:

1. In a small saucepan warm the oil over low heat.

2. Add the chopped vanilla bean, cover, and allow to steep for 1 hour.

3. Remove from the heat and strain. It's all right if you see tiny brown specks in your oil. That's just the vanilla bean seeds — they're harmless. Save the vanilla bean for other uses.

4. Add the oil back to the pan and add the beeswax, cocoa butter, and lanolin and heat until just melted.

5. Remove from the heat and stir in essential oil if you desire. If left plain, it will smell like white chocolate, sweet and yummy!

To use: Scoop out approximately 1 teaspoon (5 ml), rub between your palms to warm and improve spreadability, then massage into each foot as necessary to keep them wonderfully moisturized and smooth.

Storage: Store in a 4-ounce (112 g) jar. No refrigeration is necessary. This butter may harden in cold weather, but will soften upon skin contact.

requires the attention of a doctor combined with a balanced, healthful diet and exercise.

Treatment: Treating the foot ailments of a diabetic is usually best left in the hands of a foot specialist — too many things could go awry if home treatment is attempted. There is one exception though: Foot specialists recommend using a good moisturizer on the feet daily to help keep any corns and calluses smooth and soft, thus heading off any potential infection caused by dry skin cracks. The Vanilla Foot Butter recipe above is one of my favorites.

Prevention: Prevention is key when dealing with diabetic feet. Here are some basic tips to remember:

- Inspect your feet daily for developing corns, calluses, blisters, or anything unusual such as color change, swelling, pain, or sores that are slow to heal. Treat minor corns and calluses immediately to prevent further development.
- Check shoes for fit and wear patterns and replace as necessary. They should never be too tight or too short, since this could further impair circulation. Never wear high heels or open-toed sandals.
- Wash your feet daily with a mild soap and warm water and make sure to completely dry between your toes. Using a blow dryer on the lowest setting does a super job of drying your feet. This is especially handy if your feet are tender and rubbing with a towel would cause discomfort. Dust with powder to keep perspiration in check.
- Don't go barefoot. Always wear shoes and loose seamless socks to avoid irritation.
- Keep feet soft by applying a thick cream every night.
- If you smoke, quit! I don't need to tell you that it contributes to poor circulation and poor health in general.
- Eat a well-balanced, high-fiber, low-fat diet.
- Finally, make exercise a daily habit.

See a Physician If: Diabetes is a serious disease and an ordinary foot problem should not be ignored; it could be life-threatening if not dealt with promptly. Attempting harsh home treatments such as cutting your calluses or corns could cause bleeding and

In a pinch you can use petroleum jelly or castor oil as softening foot treatments. If you'd like a product in an elegant tube to carry in your purse or stash in an office drawer, I recommend Elizabeth Arden's Eight Hour Cream. It's a bit expensive, but conveniently sized and doubles as an excellent lip gloss, cuticle conditioner, and nail buffing cream. It's been a popular product for many, many years.

should **never** be performed. Even using a pumice stone too aggressively could open the gate for infection. Your best and safest bet is to visit a foot specialist.

Dry, Cracked Feet

Causes: Dry skin can affect any part of the body, but the soles of your feet are very susceptible because they, like the palms of your hands, lack sebaceous (oil) glands to help keep them lubricated. These glands secrete sebum, which helps prevent the evaporation of moisture from the skin.

Years ago when I worked as an aesthetician and reflexologist in a salon, I observed many pairs of dry, cracked, scaly feet and was frequently asked to recommend or formulate a lotion or cream to aid in healing the condition. Dry skin can be the result of a nutritional deficiency (specifically vitamins A, B complex, C, D, or E) or just simple neglect. Rubbing lotion on your feet every day may help a bit, but basic foot care must become a daily habit.

Symptoms: I'm assuming that the dryness and cracks on your feet aren't caused by athlete's foot. If so, then treat accordingly. So that leaves us with neglect! If you ignore your feet and the types of shoes you stick them into, then an unpleasant situation can develop: rough, dry, sometimes painful, skin. Calluses can form on your heels, balls of your feet, and on your toes. They can thicken, then crack and harden if not pared down and softened. I've got a friend whose feet become so leatherlike and fissured in winter that sometimes she can barely walk because they hurt so much.

If you exercise, your feet perspire a lot. In the warmer months this does not pose a problem, but in winter, the air is drier and colder, and your soft, sweaty feet will dry and crack after removing your running shoes if you don't care for them properly.

Simply walking around barefoot a lot or wearing open-toed sandals can lead to dry skin on your feet. Your poor dogs need some type of barrier protection between you and the drying environment, be it lotion, cream, oil, or salve.

Treatment: If you've allowed your feet to become hard and leathery, you must first soften them before you can begin healing the dry skin condition. Try the Mineral Rich Oatmeal Soak on page 147 — it's very soothing!

Prevention: Don't wait until the dead of winter to start treating your painful, leathery feet; start at summer's end with some preventative maintenance so you never reach the dreaded skin-splitting stage.

See a Physician If: If the skin on your feet has become so hard, dry, and thick that it is resistant to home treatment, a foot specialist can file or pare down the buildup so you can then proceed with proper maintenance. If your feet have developed deep fissures, become inflamed, or bleed, see a doctor to prevent infection from setting in.

The elderly, in particular, often suffer from dry skin problems, mainly due to the inability to simply bend over and reach their feet to take care of them. A doctor or perhaps a nail technician would be of great help with basic foot care needs.

SUPER RICH, ALL-PURPOSE FOOT CREAM

Here's a recipe for the thickest cream I've ever made. It's got real staying power and will keep your feet the softest they've ever been. Guaranteed! It also doubles as a fantastic lip balm and dynamite cuticle conditioner.

3   tablespoons (45 ml) plus 1 teaspoon (5 ml) castor oil
2   teaspoons (10 ml) beeswax
15 drops peppermint essential oil
15 drops rosemary essential oil

Yield: approximately ¼ cup (60 ml)

To make:
1. Over very low heat, blend the castor oil and beeswax in a small saucepan, and heat until the wax is just melted. Remove from burner and allow to cool a bit.
2. Add the essential oil drops to the bottom of a 2-ounce (55 g) jar, then pour in the oil/wax mixture.

To use:
1. Apply enough of this wonderfully thick cream to your feet each night so that your ankles are covered as well. Put on socks.
2. In the morning, apply a dab to the dryest areas before getting dressed. I usually use this formula, or a similar one, every day or so for 8 months out of the year and find that from May through August a lighter cream will suffice.

MINERAL RICH OATMEAL SOAK

If you do this procedure every other day or so you will eventually and safely remove most of the hard skin on your feet and can then reduce the treatment to 2 times per week as maintenance. This footbath feels particularly good because of the oatmeal's moisturizing and softening properties.

1 footbath tub
1/2 cup (120 ml) very finely ground oatmeal
1/4 cup (60 ml) white cosmetic clay
5 drops geranium, lavender, or eucalyptus essential oil (optional)
Pumice stone or foot file

Yield: 1 treatment

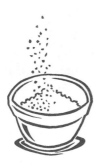

To make:

1. To make the ground oatmeal, put about ¾ cup (180 ml) old-fashioned "grocery store" variety oatmeal into a food processor and process until the oats are of a powderlike consistency.

2. Place a towel on the floor in front of the chair where you will be sitting as you soak your feet. Pour enough water into the tub (whatever temperature you desire) so that your ankles will be covered. Slowly stir in the oatmeal and clay until dissolved, then add essential oil if you desire.

To use:

1. Soak your feet for at least 10 to 15 minutes or until your calluses are soft, but not until your feet are "pruny."

2. Very gently scrub your calluses and/or corns with the pumice stone or file just until the top layer of tough dead skin has been removed.

3. Rinse, then roughly dry with a coarse towel.

4. Apply a heavy cream and put on socks.

Caution: Diabetics should not soak their feet. Most suffer from circulatory disorders and cannot feel if the water temperature is too hot or cold. Additionally, if the foot skin gets too soft as a result of soaking, it can lead to pre-ulcerations especially between the toes in the web spaces.

Hammertoes

Causes: Hammertoe, sometimes called claw toe or mallet toe, can occur in the second, third, or fourth toe, though generally the second toe is most commonly affected. This deformity is caused by shoes that are too short and tight, or narrow and pointed. Hammertoes can also be caused as a result of a bunion, which slants the big toe toward and under the second toe, thus pushing the toe up and making it virtually useless. Some contracted toes are caused by muscle imbalances, birth defects, injury, or arthritis, but most are due to ill-fitting shoes.

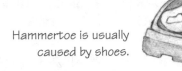

Hammertoe is usually caused by shoes.

Symptoms: The tendons contract and joints become deformed as the toe is forced back by ill-fitting shoes. The toe(s) then assume a hook or clawlike position and occasionally even cross over each other in an attempt to find more space in the crowded shoe.

To compound the problem, two additional foot maladies can accompany hammertoes. A callus usually forms under the metatarsal head and a hard corn forms on top of the bend in the toe where it rubs against your shoe. Soft corns can also form between the toes where the skin is pinched. It's an ugly situation and it hurts!

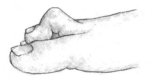

Hammertoe

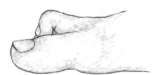

Claw toe

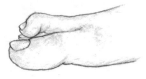

Mallet toe

FOOT FACT

Women are the most frequent sufferers of hammertoes. In fact, the American Orthopaedic Foot and Ankle Society says that women have about ninety percent of all surgeries for common foot problems, such as bunions and hammertoes. Their fashionable footwear is not wide enough in the toe box and often not long enough to allow freedom of movement. Instead their narrow, short shoes squeeze and jam the toes and ball of the foot to the point that the toes have no choice except to curl or "hammer" in an effort to try to find room for each toe to fit into the tip of the shoe.

Treatment: The treatment is easy: either modify the shoes you're wearing or modify the toes via surgery. You decide. Surgery, shoes, surgery, shoes . . . the decision shouldn't be too difficult, but it is to some people. Many would rather suffer from the deforming effects of ill-fitting shoes and be fashionably in style than wear more accommodating shoes and be pain free.

The proper shoe to wear if you have hammertoes is one with a deep toe box and a rounded shape like the toes and of a soft composition. It should be wider in the forefoot than the heel and higher in the toe box, not flat as most shoes.

Prevention: Wear shoes that fit! Stand on a piece of paper and trace your foot. Take that tracing to the shoe store and find a shoe that is a tiny bit wider and a half inch longer than your drawing. Make sure it has a snug, relatively low heel. Try those on for size. Bet you don't like them, do you? But your feet do! Keep looking — I'm sure you'll find something aesthetically appealing.

See a Physician If: If your hammertoe problem persists despite altering shoe style and relieving the pressure on the toe joints, surgery may be an option. It can reduce the prominence of the toe where the corn is formed. Your foot specialist can remove part of the bone, which will allow the toe to lie flat in the shoe.

Heel Spurs

Causes: The plantar fascia is a band of connective tissue that runs from the base of the heel to the base of the toes. Heel spurs begin when a partial separation occurs between this tissue and the heel bone. This injury may cause new bone growth in the affected area that projects out into the flesh of the foot. Other causes of heel spurs might be obesity, running, jogging, or jumping up and down in aerobics class, standing on your feet all day, wearing worn out shoes, and so forth. Anything that constantly strains the muscles that support your foot can lead to the formation of a spur.

Symptoms: A heel spur can feel like you have a rock permanently wedged in your heel or a painful bruise. The pain is most intense immediately after a period of rest, just when you begin to walk again. Actually, the more you walk, the better it feels, up to a point. Continued walking and long periods of standing will cause the heel to become quite tender.

Treatment: The painful inflammation in your heel needs to be relieved by resting your foot and applying heat with either a heating pad or hot water foot soaks to rev up the circulation, ease the pain, and reduce the swelling. When wearing shoes, place a half-inch-thick heel pad in your shoe to help cushion the pain and absorb shock. Arch supports may help to take some of the weight off your heel.

Prevention: Feet need to be stretched and allowed to relax throughout the day. If possible, remove your shoes several times a day and point and flex your feet for as long as you can and rotate your ankles. This relieves the pressure and tension on the plantar fascia.

By all means wear comfortable shoes. A firmer, motion-control shoe with a snug heel fit and ample padding in the heel area is recommended, especially if your job demands that you be on your feet a lot or you're an avid exerciser.

See a Physician If: If at-home therapy and heel padding doesn't help, your doctor may want to use steroid injections for temporary relief or may decide to make custom orthotics, which will redistribute your weight so that your foot is correctly balanced and the pressure is taken off the spur. As a last resort, your doctor can perform surgery to remove the spur (frequently this is done right in the office).

Hot Feet

Causes: There are lots of causes for hot feet, such as stress, anxiety, insufficient water intake, walking barefoot on hot pavement or beach sand, shoes and socks that are too heavy for the season, or standing all day.

Symptoms: Having hot feet is not a serious threat to your health, just a nuisance. If your feet are hot, then usually so is the rest of you, and uncomfortable to boot! Many times the symptom of hot feet is combined with itchiness, profuse sweating, and/or odor, but we'll address those individually later. I just want to show you how you can bring relief to your firey feet and cool the rest of your body simultaneously.

Treatment: My very active eighty-seven-year-old grandfather tends a large garden and raises cattle. I think his only complaints in life are his weather-sensitive, arthritic knees and his hot feet. Georgia summers can get quite sultry, so he cools his feet by soaking them daily in cool water and adds a few spoonfuls of his favorite medicinal footbath powder that contains camphor and eucalyptus. (Then he promptly falls asleep!) You could try this too, but instead of powder, add a few drops each of camphor, eucalyptus, and peppermint essential oils.

Prevention: Here are a few tips to help keep your feet cool and fresh at all times:

- Wash feet at least once but maybe twice a day with cool water, using a peppermint or tea tree essential oil soap. Try September's Sun Herbal Soap Company's "Mad about Mint" or their "Tea Tree Foot Soap" (see resources on page 177). Don't forget to dry between your toes.
- Use a mint or menthol-based foot powder liberally morning and night to keep feet delightfully dry.
- Wear comfortable, roomy shoes with light, airy socks so feet can breathe.
- Drink plenty of water.
- If you must stand all day, try to slip off your shoes every hour or so and prop your feet up. If that's not possible, remove your shoes and simply wiggle your toes and rotate your ankles for a bit of exercise.
- Take your shoes, socks, and/or hosiery off as soon as you get home and go barefoot for the rest of the evening if you can. Feet need to feel the cool ground beneath them for as many hours as possible each day.

See a Physician If: If your feet are not cooling down by using any of the above treatments and are hot *and* itchy, rashy, or developing dry skin cracks, you should probably visit a foot specialist to rule out athlete's foot, an allergy, or a rash like poison oak/ivy.

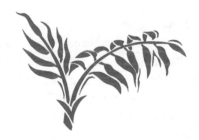

FOOT FACT

The average temperature inside your shoes is 106°F. It's a wonder your feet don't just quit and go on strike!

ROSEMARY AND PEPPERMINT COOLING LEG AND FOOT GEL

A couple of years ago, I created a fabulous herbal gel formula to use as a facial cleanser for dry, sensitive skin. It occurred to me while writing this section that it could double as a super cooling leg and foot gel, too. It leaves legs and feet feeling comfortably cool and moisturized. Contrary to what you might think, it leaves minimal residue and sinks right in. It's excellent to use after shaving your legs.

1 teaspoon (5 ml) finely powdered marshmallow root
1 tablespoon (15 ml) water
2 drops peppermint essential oil
2 drops rosemary or eucalyptus essential oil

Yield: 1 treatment

To make: In a small bowl, stir together all ingredients until a tan-colored, thick, speckled, slippery gel forms. This will happen very quickly.

To use: Apply 1 teaspoon (5 ml) of this gel to each leg and foot and massage in until the gel is no longer slippery.

Storage: Cover and refrigerate any leftovers for up to 3 days.

Note: To make the gel especially refreshing, chill for 1 hour prior to use.

ON YOUR FEET ALL DAY: A CAREER TIP

In 1987, while in school training for my aesthetician license, my instructors stressed this point over and over again, "Give your feet a few minutes' daily care. It's essential to good posture and good health. Healthy feet help produce a more pleasing personality."

Initially, I didn't understand how taking care of my feet affected my personality. After I'd worked in a salon for a while, it became clear. Standing eight hours a day in fashionable shoes hurts! Anyone who works on his or her feet all day knows that if your feet are constantly hurting, you feel miserable. It's much easier to smile and be cheerful with comfortable, cared-for feet.

MINT CHILLER FOOT LOTION

You've probably seen, if not used, the popular pink peppermint foot lotions sold by a few bath and body shops located in malls nationwide. They usually sell for approximately twenty dollars for a 16-ounce (454-g) bottle. That seems pretty pricey to me! Here's how to make your own for a fraction of the price. Mine smells more invigorating and minty, too, and it's super refreshing!

½ cup (120 ml) almond or soybean oil

1 tablespoon (15 ml) beeswax

½ teaspoon (2 ml) borax

⅓ cup (80 ml) plus 1 tablespoon (15 ml) warm, strong peppermint tea

3 drops red or green food coloring (optional)

½ teaspoon (2 ml) peppermint or spearmint essential oil

Yield: 1 cup (230 ml)

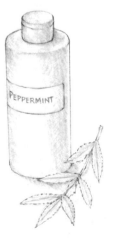

To make:

1. In a small pan over very low heat, melt the oil and wax.

2. In another saucepan, stir the borax into the warm tea until completely dissolved, and add food coloring if desired. (The peppermint tea can be made by simply pouring a cup of boiling water over a peppermint tea bag or 1 teaspoon [5 ml] of the dried herb, steeping for 5 to 10 minutes, then straining and cooling a bit.)

3. The two mixtures should be approximately the same temperature before you perform the next step. While whisking vigorously with your small whisk, slowly drizzle the warm tea/borax liquid into the oil/wax mixture, then add the essential oil. The cream will begin to thicken and should have a lotion-like consistency. If you place the oil/wax pan in a bowl of ice while whisking, the lotion will set up much faster.

To use: Massage into legs and feet anytime they need a little revitalizing. Keep the lotion in the refrigerator in the summer for an extra chilling sensation!

Storage: Store in a plastic squeeze bottle or decorative glass bottle. Use within thirty days, or sooner if weather is hot.

Ingrown Toenails

Causes: Ingrown toenails are nails that have become imbedded in the surrounding soft flesh of the toe. The big toe is most often affected, but the other toes can also suffer.

This painful condition can be caused by wearing short, tight shoes, socks, or hosiery; poor nail care; injury to the nail bed; fungus; and heredity. Obese people are particularly susceptible, too. Their feet gain weight just like the rest of the body and the skin can swell up and around the toenail. Combine this with the excess pressure placed upon the feet, and a bit of improper nail clipping, and you've got a recipe for pain.

Most ingrown toenails are self-inflicted. If you rip off your toenails with your fingers instead of cutting them, you leave jagged edges, which dig into the nail groove when your tight shoe presses against the toenail. Improper clipping by cutting the nail too short and rounding the corners can cause the same problem.

Symptoms: An infection called *paronychia* can result when the toenail penetrates the flesh. It begins as minor swelling, redness, and clear fluid oozing from the site. If ignored, it can become infected, very painful and swollen. Walking at this point is unbearable. If still left untreated, pus will exude from the infected site and red streaks can appear along the foot and shoot up the leg. The infection is dangerous now and can enter the bloodstream, causing you to become ill, possibly leading to the loss of a toe, foot, or leg if gangrene sets in. This, thankfully, is a rare occurrence.

Treatment: To treat an ingrown toenail in its beginning stages, soak your foot in a foot tub filled with warm, strong sage and yarrow tea (make this by using ¼ cup [60 ml] of each dried herb per gallon of boiling water, then steep, strain, and cool until comfortable), ½ cup (120 ml) of sea salt, and a few drops of tea tree or lavender essential oil for 10 to 15 minutes. Dry thoroughly. Now, take a sliver of cotton and using a toothpick, ever so gently wedge the cotton under the offending toenail. Leave it there until the nail grows out. It will help direct the nail's growth over the skin. Apply a drop of thyme, lavender, or tea tree essential oil on the site daily to help keep infection at bay.

> **FOOT FACT**
>
> Ten percent of Americans have had an ingrown toenail at one time or another. It is the most common toenail impairment.

Prevention: Try these tips to help prevent the occurrence of this painful affliction:

- Clip toenails straight across so that they are just about even with the tip of the toe and file any pointed edges smooth with an emery board.
- Examine your feet daily after washing and drying to nip any potential problems in the bud.
- Wear comfortable shoes and socks. Shoes and/or hosiery should never constrict your feet.

See a Physician If: If you're diabetic, don't allow a minor foot malady to become potentially life-threatening; see a foot specialist immediately. For an infection, antibiotics may be prescribed to clear it up. If an ingrown toenail is a recurrent problem, your doctor may want to perform a *matrixectomy* (removal of the germinal matrix, the source of nail growth, along with the edge of the nail plate). This is a permanent narrowing of the toenail.

FOOT FACT

Ingrown toenails most often occur in children, teens, and young adults, primarily because they don't heed early warning signs that something is amiss. Also, young people's feet grow so fast that they frequently wear shoes that are too short, tight, or worn out, which puts pressure and friction on the edges of the toenails. Foot health is not uppermost in their thoughts at this age either. Toenails are often not cut properly and feet are basically neglected. This is why it's essential that you examine your child's feet every day and instill the importance of proper foot care.

Itchy Feet

Causes: Itchy feet can have a myriad of causes, including ringworm, athlete's foot, an allergy to socks or hosiery, detergent, soap, or lotion, poison oak or poison ivy, eczema, psoriasis, simple dry skin, or a nutritional deficiency of unsaturated fatty acids. *Candida albicans* (yeastlike fungi) can cause the whole body to itch.

From: _____

BUSINESS REPLY MAIL

FIRST-CLASS MAIL   PERMIT NO. 2   POWNAL VT

POSTAGE WILL BE PAID BY ADDRESSEE

STOREY'S BOOKS FOR COUNTRY LIVING
STOREY COMMUNICATIONS INC
RR1 BOX 105
POWNAL VT   05261-9988

We'd love your thoughts . . .

Your reactions, criticisms, things you did or didn't like about this Storey Book. Please use space below (or write a letter if you'd prefer — even send photos!) telling how you've made use of the information . . . how you've put it to work . . . the more details the better!

Thanks in advance for your help in building our library of good Storey Books.

Pamela B. Art

Publisher, Storey Books

Book Title: _____

Purchased From: _____

Comments: _____

_____

_____

_____

_____

Your Name: _____

Mailing Address: _____

_____

E-mail Address: _____

☐ Please check here if you'd like our latest Storey's Books for Country Living Catalog.

☐ You have my permission to quote from my comments and use these quotations in ads, brochures, mail, and other promotions used to market Storey Books.

Signed _____ Date _____

e-mail=feedback@storey.com   www.storey.com   PRINTED IN THE USA   4/98

Symptoms: Feet that itch are annoying. Sometimes they're hot and tingly and other times they just need a good scratching. Unlike your arm or your nose, you can't scratch your feet every time you have the urge. They can make you feel miserable.

Treatment: The Moisturizing Anti-Itch Foot Formula below is my two-step treatment for keeping your feet itch-free, fungus-free, and velvety soft.

Prevention: Try these tips to help prevent itchy feet:

- ◆ Switch to natural fiber socks/hosiery and open-toed shoes so your feet can breathe. Synthetic fibers and snug-fitting shoes trap moisture and heat that can lead to itchy feet.
- ◆ Moisturize feet daily. Dry air causes feet to lose elasticity and natural oils, which results in dry skin and cracking. Dry skin itches!
- ◆ Apply powder to your feet and shoes every day. Try the Happy Feet recipe on page 121 to help keep fungus at bay.

See a Physician If: If the above treatment or prevention measures fail, visit your foot specialist. He or she may want to rule out a fungus infection or other skin disease.

MOISTURIZING ANTI-ITCH FOOT FORMULA

1 teaspoon (5 ml) walnut hulls

1 cup (230 ml) water

3 tablespoons (45 ml) Calendula Blossom Oil (see recipe on page 132)

10 drops tea tree essential oil

5 drops eucalyptus essential oil

Yield: approximately 1 ¼ cups (290 ml)

1. Simmer walnut hulls in water for 30 minutes, strain. Pour ½ cup (120 ml) of tea over feet and massage in real well, including between your toes. Pat dry (use a dark towel, as the tea will stain lighter colored ones). Store excess in refrigerator for up to 5 days.

2. Blend Calendula Blossom Oil with tea tree and eucalyptus essential oils. After following step 1, rub 1 teaspoon of this oil formula in thoroughly. Put on socks. Store remainder in refrigerator, tightly covered, for up to 1 year.

Metatarsalgia

Causes: The causes of this painful malady are many. Women suffer more frequently than men, due to their high-heeled, narrow shoes. Wearing high heels puts added pressure on the metatarsal heads. Plus, if the shoes are too narrow, this can put pressure on the anterior metatarsal arch. This arch normally flexes up and down as you walk, but if the shoes you're wearing are too tight and the ends of the arch are made rigid, no longer flexible, the result may be that one or more of the metatarsals drops out of alignment. When this happens, the bones are brought closer to the surface and can easily become bruised, callused, and inflamed.

If you've got high-arched feet, thin feet without much fat padding and prominent bones, or if you put lots of mileage on your feet from sports activities, you may be susceptible to metatarsalgia. Anything that causes you to come down hard on your metatarsals can lead to pain in this area.

Symptoms: According to my Taber's Cyclopedic Medical Dictionary, metatarsalgia is a severe pain or cramp in the anterior portion of the metatarsus. In other words, pain occurs under your metatarsal heads or, simply put, in your forefoot region. It can feel as if you've got a pebble in your shoe or a bruised bone in the ball of your foot.

Treatment: Since one or more of the metatarsal heads is depressed, you need to elevate it. Using a ¼-inch (.6-cm) thick piece of felt or rubber, cut it into a 2- to 3-inch (5- to 7.6-cm) long strip by approximately 2 inches (5 cm) wide (depending on the size of your foot), and tape it behind your metatarsal heads.

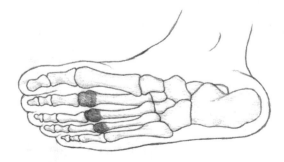

The darkened area shows where pain occurs with metatarsalgia.

Where are your metatarsal heads and how do you know which one(s) is actually causing the pain? Gently pull your toes up and back and feel the area where the toes connect to the metatarsal bones. Take your thumb and push up under each metatarsal bone until you find the spot(s) that makes you grimace, if not scream from the pain. You want to put your padding behind this area, in the direction of the heel.

A sporting goods store or better drugstore will carry commercial metatarsal pads or bars. Sometimes a full-length arch support is available with metatarsal pads built right in. These might be helpful.

Foot exercises such as picking up towels, marbles, or pencils with your toes can strengthen the anterior metatarsal arch, as well as stretch and relax your feet.

Prevention: Follow these tips to keep your feet pain free:

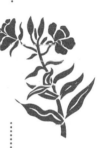

- ◆ Women, listen up: you need to lower your heels and wear roomier shoes. If you insist on wearing high heels, find one of the more recent shoe innovations for working women, a "comfort" pump (a marketing oxymoron) that has plenty of built-in forefoot padding and arch support, though it's still not wide enough in the toe box.
- ◆ Wear well-cushioned shoes with super soft midsoles and plenty of room in the toe box. Add cushioned insoles with arch supports, if necessary.
- ◆ If you're an avid exerciser, please wear proper shoes with thick socks and don't wear your shoes beyond their lifespan, or you'll end up with cushioning that's shot and insufficient padding (see chapter 5, What's Afoot? Selecting Proper Footwear) to protect your foot from landing too hard.

See a Physician If: Usually metatarsalgia will respond to a change in shoe environment or to appropriate padding. If you're still experiencing pain, a foot specialist may recommend a custom orthotic to redistribute the weight on your foot. Steroid injections may sometimes be used to help reduce any inflammation. Surgery is a last resort if your foot doesn't respond to conservative care. The offending metatarsal bone can be cut off, reducing the prominence.

Morton's Foot

Causes: You've probably seen plenty of people who have feet in which the second toe is longer than the big toe. It's sometimes referred to as Morton's syndrome foot (so named after Dr. Dudley J. Morton in the 1930s) and it's relatively commonplace. For once, I'm not going to blame this condition on shoes. Instead, blame your parents. It's genetic.

You can't always tell just by looking that you have Morton's foot; it's not that obvious in some people. Your doctor would know by looking at an X ray. Actually, the problem is not that the second toe is extra long, it's the first metatarsal bone that the big toe is attached to that's short.

Symptoms: Morton's foot causes pain to develop in the ball of your foot, such as in a condition called *second metatarsal phalangeal inflammation*, in which the base of the metatarsal becomes inflamed and painful. Calluses can develop under the second toe, and the other toes can become hammertoes with corns on top.

Under normal conditions, as you're walking, your big toe will be the first to reach where you're going. But, with a Morton's foot, it's the second toe that hits first. It suffers more ligament disruption and bangs into things. It's not as strong as the big toe. When you run and walk, you're supposed to push off with your big toe, but because the metatarsal is shorter in this case, it can't quite perform it's job as well as it should, so the second toe has to carry some of the weight. This causes a weight shift which can lead to leg, knee, hip, and spinal misalignment problems.

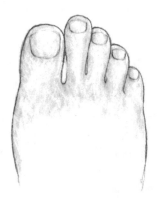

Morton's foot

Treatment: It's not the short first toe that receives treatment; it's the resulting problems that do: calluses, corns, hammertoes, and metatarsal pain. See previous descriptions on how to treat these individually.

Prevention: Since Morton's foot is a "gift" from Mother Nature, you can't prevent it as you can other afflictions. The key is to help prevent the secondary problems from occurring. Foot specialists suggest wearing a stiff-soled shoe that's stiff in the forefoot to cut down on motion. A cross trainer or court shoe works well. Don't wear a running shoe; it's too soft and flexible in the toe box.

See a Physician If: If you'd rather trade your Morton's foot for another that's more to your liking, a foot specialist may be able to create a custom soft orthotic for you that will raise the head of the first metatarsal and give you more forefoot control. This will help with the misalignment problems you're probably suffering from, too.

FOOT FACT

The skin on the sole of your foot is the thickest on the body — three times thicker than the skin on your palms and fifteen times thicker than your delicate facial skin. The plantar fat pad thins as you age. Certain disease states, such as rheumatoid arthritis and diabetes, also cause this padding to atrophy.

Neuroma

Causes: A neuroma is a tumor composed of nerve cells, usually occurring between the third and fourth metatarsal heads, but it can occur in the others. It is caused by compression or irritation of the nerves as a result of improper footwear or overpronation.

Symptoms: A neuroma feels like fiery, shooting, stabbing pain or tingling and numbness reaching out into your toes. The pain and discomfort can come and go at will. Once again, this is a foot problem that most often affects women's feet.

Overpronation of the foot, or too much inward rolling, results in a "looser" forefoot; in other words, your metatarsal bones have more movement, more play. This excess movement irritates the nerves that run between the metatarsal heads, eventually causing them to become inflamed and quite painful.

Treatment: When you feel a sudden shooting, burning, stabbing pain in this region of your forefoot, remove your shoes immediately and massage your foot. Relieving your foot of shoe compression often brings quick relief. If possible, give your foot some ice treatment as soon as the pain begins by setting your foot on a bag of ice for five to ten minutes, then off for five to ten. Do this three or four times. Repeat several times per week. It will help relieve some of the inflammation. Of course, the pain *will* keep coming back if you continue to wear shoes that squeeze your foot, and if left untreated, it can become excruciating, so much so that walking becomes unbearable.

If the pain is caused by an overpronating foot, you need to wear motion-controlled shoes. The rear foot and forefoot need stability; make sure the toe box is wide enough so as not to compress your bones.

Prevention: "Cruel and inhumane" — that pretty much sums up the consensus of foot specialists if asked to describe high-heeled, pointed-toe shoes. They seem to be the cause of so many foot problems. Men's narrow-toed, snug leather shoes are guilty, too, but not to the same degree. Neuromas can be prevented by not wearing this type of shoe, but if you insist on making a fashion statement, despite the discomfort afforded by these shoes, take them off frequently during the day and only wear them once or twice per week. Better still, find some fashionable, comfortable shoes and give your feet a break for a change!

See a Physician If: If changing your shoe environment doesn't help, and this is a long-standing problem, a foot specialist can use steroid injection therapy to calm the neuroma. Orthotics are frequently prescribed to give more arch support and elevate and reduce the motion of the metatarsal heads, thus lessening the irritation. As a last resort, in severe cases, surgery is performed to remove the tumor (scar tissue that has developed around the irritated nerve).

Odoriferous and Sweaty Feet

Causes: Think back a few decades ago (depending on your age) to Halloween night. Do you remember running up to the neighbor's door, all dressed up in your scariest costume, and yelling, "Trick or treat, smell my feet, give me something good to eat?" I realize it was all said in jest, but I can guarantee your neighbor wouldn't find that such a "treat" if you really made them smell your feet! All kidding aside, foot odor, or plantar bromidrosis, can be a seriously embarrassing physical as well as psychological problem for some people. It is caused by an overabundance of foot perspiration and bacteria.

The rate of sweat production is greatly affected by a wide range of emotions such as fear, nervousness, falling in love, and performance anxiety, be it sexual or on-the-job stress. Drinking lots of water, exercising heavily, working at a physically demanding job, or wearing tight-fitting shoes or shoes made of nonbreathable materials for extended periods of time will also cause your feet to sweat. Some people have a genetic predisposition to foot odor and wetness, which tends to run in families.

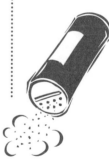

Symptoms: When moisture and bacteria comingle inside a pair of shoes, they can create such an overwhelming stench that the poor sufferer will avoid social occasions and even shopping for new shoes. Excessive perspiration will cause destruction of footwear as the stitching, construction materials, and padding breakdown prematurely from the constant pressure and moisture within.

Foot odor is "unique and, next to alcoholic breath, may be the most distinctive scent in the office setting. It's often described as musty, amino-like, cheesy, or rancid," says Walter J. Pedowitz, M.D.

Treatment: You know when your feet stink, unless you suffer from odor perception deficit. There are people who actually can't discern a sweet fragrance from stink (poor souls) and some who have gotten so used to the way their feet smell that they no longer notice the unpleasantness, but everyone around them does! Hopefully, if you suffer from this smelly affliction you will try some of my remedies to fix this distressful, air-fouling problem.

Prevention: Follow these tips for fresh feet:

◆ First and foremost, wash and dry your feet once or twice daily. Proper hygiene is imperative!
◆ Increase your chlorophyll intake. Spirulina, parsley, and green drinks are high in vitamin A and chlorophyll, which is a known internal odor fighter.
◆ Alternate shoes each day to allow for a 24-hour dry out period between wearings.
◆ Sprinkle baking soda into your shoes after you take them off for the evening to help absorb moisture and odor.
◆ If you're prone to foot odor, avoid strong foods such as garlic, onions, certain cheeses, black pepper, and eggs.
◆ Wear baking soda impregnated, cushioned insoles in your shoes and change them often.
◆ Make sure hose, shoes, and socks are made of natural fibers, fit properly, and allow your feet to breathe.
◆ Change socks or hosiery twice a day if necessary and reapply powder to keep feet super dry and prevent soggy skin.
◆ Underarm antiperspirant can be applied to the soles of your feet as well. It works for some people by lessening the amount of sweat produced and preventing bacterial growth. If you'd like to try this approach, I recommend using a natural brand first. Health food stores carry various herbal-based brands sans chemicals.

See a Physician If: If your condition is not responding to any of the above measures, a foot specialist may want to administer a topical antibiotic or recommend daily soaks with potassium permanganate to decrease odor production. Other drugs such as tranquilizers to soothe a nervous disposition or topical scented formaldehyde can be prescribed, but can have terrible side effects and should be avoided if at all possible. Diseases such as hyperthyroidism, hypoadrenalism, anemia, and thermoregulatory disturbances can cause profuse sweating, too, and should be ruled out.

ODOR AWAY REFRESHING FOOT SPRAY

1 cup (230 ml) commercial witch hazel or ½ cup (120 ml) of your homemade witch hazel tincture added to ½ cup (120 ml) distilled water (see Witch Hazel Tincture recipe on page 43)

20 drops spearmint or peppermint essential oil

40 drops geranium essential oil

Yield: 1 cup (230 ml)

To make: Pour all ingredients into an 8-ounce decorative spray bottle. Shake well.
To use: Spray feet any time they need cooling and revitalizing. Best to use if you're not going to be wearing shoes for the next hour or so, so feet can dry naturally. This allows the astringent properties of the witch hazel and the cooling, deodorizing, and antimicrobial properties of the essential oils to go about their duties.
Storage: Refrigeration is not necessary. Use within one year for maximum potency.

WHITE OAK REMEDY

The following remedy was actually recommended in 1883 by J.I. Lighthall, the Great Indian Medicine Man, in his book, *The Indian Household Medicine Guide.* "There is no tree better known than the White Oak, nor is there a tree more useful to mankind. It grows in all parts of the United States. There are three kinds of Oaks: the red, the white, and the black. The inner bark is the part used as a medicine, and a very good one it is, too.

"**Medicinal properties and uses:** The bark is a powerful astringent. It makes a splendid wash for old sores and wounds when mattering and not inclined to heal. The best form to use it in is a strong tea made from the green bark. It will cure bad smelling and sweaty feet by washing them with it."

ODOR NEUTRALIZING ORANGE FOOT POWDER

Foot odor has more than just one symptom. It is frequently accompanied by soggy skin, blisters, tenderness between the toes, and susceptibility to fungus and infection. This powder will help to absorb the odor, keep your feet dry, and fight fungus (if you add the tea tree and thyme essential oils or geranium essential oil). Orange essential oil is a terrific odor fighter!

½ cup (120 ml) baking soda
½ cup (120 ml) arrowroot
2 tablespoons (30 ml) zinc oxide powder
2 tablespoons (30 ml) fine, white clay
1 teaspoon (5 ml) orange or geranium essential oil (both do a great job!)
½ teaspoon (2 ml) tea tree essential oil (optional)
½ teaspoon (2 ml) thyme essential oil (optional)

Yield: approximately 1¼ cups (290 ml)

To make: Mix dry ingredients in a large bowl or food processor. Add the essential oils a few drops at a time and thoroughly incorporate into powder.

To use: Sprinkle into shoes and socks once or twice daily.

Storage: Store this in a special shaker container or recycle a plastic spice jar (not one that previously held dried onions or garlic, though). Refrigeration is not necessary. Use within one year for maximum potency.

Plantar Warts

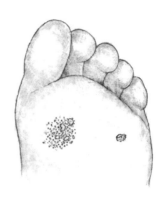

Causes: A *verruca plantaris*, or plantar wart, appears on the plantar surface or sole of your foot and is caused by an easily transmittable virus. You can just as easily transmit it to other parts of your body or to someone else. Just like athlete's foot fungus, the virus can be contracted by walking bare foot in warm, moist environments such as in gyms, locker rooms, saunas, showers, pool areas, and public bathrooms. Cracks or abrasions on your feet are an open invitation for the virus to go deep inside the dermal layers and take up residence. Scratching or shaving over the affected area can also spread the infection.

Symptoms: The wart can range in size from a tiny dot to the size of a nickel or larger and appear singly or in clusters, but can easily be confused with a callus or corn because the warts are covered with thick skin tissue. A plantar wart, though, has a distinct black or brown pinpoint in the center, which is the site of a blood vessel, and will hurt if you squeeze it and bleed if you cut it; a corn will not. These warts occur most frequently on the balls and heels of the feet.

Plantar warts can be quite painful and become pushed deep inside the skin due to weight and shoe pressure.

A mosaic wart is caused by the same virus, is irregular in shape and bleeds easily when irritated, and can eventually form a large cluster of a hundred or more tiny warts. This patch of warts can cover the entire bottom of the foot and has a rougher, thicker surface than a plantar wart.

Treatment: A cure for these pesky, painful growths can be elusive at best because they frequently go away spontaneously and also tend to recur spontaneously in the same areas. There is no guaranteed cure, natural or chemical. Just when you think they're gone, here they come again.

FOOT FACT

The American Podiatric Medical Association says that, "Children, especially teenagers, tend to be more susceptible to warts than adults; some people seem to be immune, and never get them."

Some foot specialists recommend the cost-effective treatment of repeatedly applying salicylic acid drops (found in the foot care section of your drugstore). File the wart down slightly with an emery board daily, apply a drop of acid, file again the next day, apply acid . . . keep treating daily for several weeks or months until the wart dissolves. Care should be taken to avoid getting this acid on the surrounding skin, as it can burn and dissolve healthy tissue as well as the wart(s).

Caution: Diabetics should never try this.

Herbal and folklore wart remedies abound. You could try applying the milky, sticky sap from a dandelion stem, calendula stem, or milkweed stem to the wart and covering with an adhesive bandage. Change dressing daily. These saps act as corrosive agents to remove the wart.

Tea tree essential oil can be applied "neat" (undiluted), as can garlic oil. These both have powerful antiviral properties. A slice of raw garlic can be taped to the affected area with a fresh piece being applied daily. Vitamin A oil is said to remove warts, too. No one treatment works for everyone. Whatever method you choose to try, keep at it. Warts can be stubborn creatures.

Prevention: Since the virus that causes plantar warts is highly contagious, please avoid going barefoot in the gym or around swimming pools, or any place that's public, warm, and moist. Wash and dry your feet daily and put powder in your shoes to absorb moisture. Also, if you are treating or inspecting someone else's infected feet, wear disposable gloves and wash your hands thoroughly.

HUMOROUS WART MYTHS

Warts do not bring on seven years of bad luck nor do you get seven years of good luck when they go away. They are not caused by frog pee-pee or by holding a frog. (I know you believed this when you were a child — I did!) You will not turn into a witch if you continue to get warts or if they spread to your nose and chin, nor can you wear a garlic necklace to ward off warts.

See a Physician If: Plantar warts are sometimes difficult to treat. If yours continue to spread and are making walking painful, see a doctor. Electric needle treatments, acid peels, freezing with dry ice, or laser surgery can be used by a foot specialist to get rid of warts. Try to avoid surgery if possible so that no painful scars are left on the bottom of your foot.

Sesamoiditis

Located under the head of the first metatarsal bone (or big toe joint) are two, possibly three or four, small bones, about the size of your pinky fingernail, that "float" in the tendon of a small muscle. By that I mean that these bones don't connect to any other bones. Their purpose is to protect the first metatarsal head from injury and absorb shock. Sesamoid bones are also found in other areas of the body where considerable pressure develops, such as in your wrist and knees.

Causes: The main causes of sesamoiditis are excessive running, dancing (as in ballet, aerobics, country and western dance) combined with wearing tight shoes. It's caused by anything you do repeatedly that causes you to pound on the ball of your foot while wearing shoes in which the toe box is not wide enough. Another cause? You simply could have thin, bony feet with insufficient fat padding on the sole that won't stand up to all the pounding they're receiving.

Symptoms: The sesamoids can become bruised, inflamed, or even fractured if the initial pain and irritation are ignored and physical activity is continued. It will feel like a pebble has permeated your foot.

How do you know you've injured your sesamoids? Bend your toes up and back towards you. Now take your thumb and push up hard just under your first metatarsal head. If you're screaming "OUCH" or some other lovely word, then you've bruised or broken your bones.

Treatment: Your feet will usually feel better immediately after you take off your narrow shoes and rub them a bit. If the pain is severe, do an ice treatment by placing your foot on an ice bag for five to ten minutes, then off for five

FOOT FACT

Active people with bunions, high-arched feet, or arthritis are frequent sufferers of sesamoiditis.

to ten, alternating for a total of three to four times. This should help bring down any inflammation. Rest your foot as often as possible, too.

For conservative treatment, a wider and stiffer shoe is recommended to restrict the range of motion in the toe area. A cross-trainer is a good type to try. You might also want to add padded inserts to cushion your forefoot or place a ¼-inch (.6-cm) triangular rubber or felt padding, with a slight v-shaped cut out, around the base of the first metatarsal head to relieve the pressure on the bones.

Prevention: If you're very active, then by all means wear the proper shoes, something comfortable and not too narrow, unless you're a ballerina; then you have no choice as to shoe type. If you suffer from a bony foot, add the appropriate padding in the forefoot area and buy shoes with sufficient padding.

See a Physician If: In most cases, sesamoiditis responds quite nicely to a change in shoe environment. If the pain is not responding to home care, a foot specialist may want to give steroid injections to relieve the pain. Your doctor might also want to make a custom orthotic to shift the excess weight away from the ball of your foot.

Sore, Achy Feet

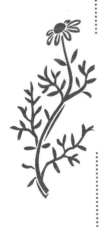

Causes: I'm pretty sure you know the cause of your sore feet. Perhaps you stand all day at work, chase your children around the house, wear fashionable shoes that don't fit properly, or work out a lot. Whatever the reason behind your pain, you want relief and you want it now!

Symptoms: "My Feet Are Killing Me!" Ever said that after being on your feet all day? Sore feet feel tired, like they've lost their "spring." Sometimes they even swell, burn, or feel tender if you've been wearing snug-fitting, blister-causing shoes.

Treatment: The following herbal recipes will help to refresh, restore, and revitalize your tired, cramped, burning, swollen dogs. They serve double duty in that they also reduce foot odor.

The following two quotes are from the book *Herbal Recipes* by Clarence Meyer (Meyerbooks, Glenwood, Illinois, 1978). It's interesting to see what types of herbal remedies were prescribed nearly two centuries ago for foot problems such as calluses, swelling, corns, or sprains.

"The bark of the root of bittersweet with chamomile and wormwood makes an ointment of great value, which is an excellent thing for a bruise, sprain, calice, swelling, or for corns" (*New Guide to Health: or, Botanic Physician,* Samuel Thomson, 1831).

"Take tansy, wormwood, horehound, catnip, and hops, of each an equal quantity. Bruise them and put them into a kettle, cover over with spirits and lard, and let it stand 2 weeks; then simmer awhile and strain. Add 1 lb. of common white turpentine to every 10 lbs. of the ointment. This ointment is very cooling, resolvent, relaxing, and emollient. It is very useful in sprains, contusions, swellings, dislocations, contracted sinews, etc." (*The American Practice of Medicine,* W. Beach, M.D., 1833).

Prevention: Sometimes daily sore feet can't be completely prevented due to job or lifestyle demands. But by wearing really comfortable shoes with shock-absorbing insoles; massaging your feet; taking soothing herbal footbaths made with yarrow, sage, thyme, or peppermint with a scoop of baking soda and Epsom salts added; and paying extra attention to foot hygiene, you should have lots of spring in your step most of the time.

See a Physician If: If your feet are chronically sore, and changing your shoe environment and trying the Sweet Relief–Aspirin for the Feet Salve treatment doesn't help alleviate some of the soreness, then see a foot specialist. He or she may want to check for misalignment problems, ingrown toenails, arthritis, bunion development, and so forth.

> If any herbe infeste the earth with its abundance, let man heed its virtues for his ills.
>
> Culpeper

SWEET RELIEF — ASPIRIN FOR THE FEET SALVE

This recipe calls for St.-John's-wort oil. To make the infused oil, see Julie Bailey's Calendula Blossom Oil recipe on page 132, but substitute St.–John's–wort flowers for the calendula blossoms. Fresh is best, but dried is okay. You can also purchase the prepared oil in better health food stores. All of the herbs in this recipe have pain-relieving properties.

½ cup (120 ml) St.-John's-wort oil

1 tablespoon (15 ml) dried meadowsweet or 2 tablespoons (30 ml) fresh flowers and leaves (wilted for 24 hours in the shade to remove excess moisture)

1 tablespoon (15 ml) powdered white willow bark

½ teaspoon (2 ml) powdered cayenne pepper

1–2 tablespoons (15–30 ml) beeswax (use the greater amount if you want a stiffer salve)

10 drops each peppermint, camphor, eucalyptus, and clove essential oils

Yield: approximately ½ cup (120 ml)

To make:
1. In a half-pint, widemouthed jar combine the St.-John's-wort oil, meadowsweet, white willow, and cayenne. Tightly seal and place in the full sun for approximately 4 weeks.
2. Shake daily.
3. Strain through hosiery or cheesecloth to remove the powder granules. Make sure to squeeze all the oil out of the straining material to get every precious drop.
4. In a small saucepan, over very low heat, melt the beeswax and stir in oil. Remove from heat and add essential oils after mixture cools a bit.
5. Pour into a decorative widemouthed plastic or glass jar.
To use: Massage a fingerful of salve into clean, tired feet as desired. This feels especially good if you can talk someone else into doing the massaging for you!
Storage: Refrigeration is not necessary. Use within six months for maximum potency.

Toenail Fungus

Causes: Ugly and embarrassing — that's how best to describe the condition of toenails infected with fungus. People with toenail fungus often avoid social situations that call for baring their feet, such as summer pool parties or strolling on the beach.

Onychomycosis is caused by microorganisms called dermatophytes, which are similar to those that cause athlete's foot. These organisms are present on your clothes and in your shoes, the gym, and even your organically fortified garden soil. They're practically unavoidable.

Symptoms: One or more of your toenails will begin to look a bit abnormal. Color changes can appear, such as long, yellowish streaks or white patches that can be scraped off. The nail can lift and begin to separate from the nail bed, thicken, and become brittle and flaky. It can also become distorted in shape and begin to twist. This fungus can be transmitted easily to your fingernails, or to other members of your family for that matter, if you constantly pick at your toes without washing your hands afterward. It sounds disgusting, but lots of people do it unintentionally.

Treatment: In order to treat toenail fungus, you have to get underneath the nail, which can be difficult. The fungus lives on the soft skin of the nail bed. The herbs and oils in the recipes on pages 174 and 175 have traditionally been used by herbalists with much success if applied at least once a day. Twice is better.

Prevention: Since toenail fungus is infectious, take the same precautions as you would with athlete's foot and wear the appropriate footwear when in public bathing places. Observe proper daily foot hygiene; keep feet fresh and dry with powder and clean changes of socks/hosiery; wear good-fitting, breathable shoes; and never trim toenails too close to the skin or cut the skin.

See a Physician If: Toenail fungus is difficult to treat. If the above measures fail, visit your foot specialist. He or she may want to prescribe a topical or oral medication to combat the fungus or perhaps remove the diseased nail, depending on the severity of the infection. Medications are not without side effects, and do not always work, either.

ANTIFUNGAL TOENAIL LINIMENT

4 tablespoons (60 ml) dried black walnut hulls or 8 tablespoons (120 ml) fresh and chopped fine

2 tablespoons (30 ml) dried, chopped goldenseal or Oregon grape root

1 tablespoon (15 ml) powdered myrrh gum

40 drops tea tree essential oil

40 drops thyme essential oil

40 drops tincture of iodine

2 cups (460 ml) vodka, brandy, rum, or gin (must be at least 80-proof or 40 percent alcohol by volume)

Yield: approximately 1½ cups (350 ml)

To make:

1. In a quart-sized (liter-sized), wide-mouthed canning jar, add the black walnut hulls, goldenseal or oregon grape root, myrrh gum, essential oils, and iodine, then pour in the alcohol. Cap tightly and store in a dark, cool place.

2. Shake daily.

3. After at least 14 days have passed (I recommend 4 to 12 weeks; it makes for a stronger formula), you may strain the mixture through hosiery-lined cheese-cloth, then squeeze and twist the cloth to wring out all the liquid.

4. Pour the finished formula into two, 8-ounce (228-g) bottles with dropper tops.

To use: Morning, noon, and night, if possible, apply a few drops to toenails, rub in thoroughly, and allow to dry before putting on hosiery, socks, or footwear. Repeat this procedure daily for as long as it takes to rid your toenails of fungus. The herbs in this recipe have potent antifungal and anti-microbial properties.

Storage: Refrigeration is not necessary. This product will keep indefinitely!

FOOT FACT

Foot specialists estimate that approximately seven to eight million people in the United States suffer from toenail fungus, but only a quarter of them seek a doctor for treatment.

TOUGH ON FUNGUS TOENAIL DROPS

You can use this recipe in conjunction with the Antifungal Toenail Liniment on the previous page. Apply this oil after the liniment has dried. Use this oil consistently for at least six months or longer or until the fungus has disappeared.

2 teaspoons (10 ml) tea tree essential oil
2 teaspoons (10 ml) thyme essential oil
2 teaspoons (10 ml) camphor essential oil
1- ounce (28-g) dropper-topped bottle

Yield: approximately 1 ounce (28 g)

To make: Combine all three essential oils and pour into the bottle. Shake well.
To use: Place a drop or two on each toenail morning and night and rub in well, then dress as you normally do.
Storage: Store in a cool, dry place.

A FINAL NOTE

Thanks for reading the book. Do you have a question? If so, I always try to personally answer all my reader mail, **but you must** enclose a self-addressed, stamped, letter-size envelope in order for me to reply. Address your letter to:

Stephanie L. Tourles
P.O. Box 772
W. Hyannisport, MA 02672

Suggested Reading

This list includes resources for this book, as well as selections from my personal library of natural health books.

Abrams, Karl J. *Algae to the Rescue!* Studio City, CA: Logan House Publications, 1996.

Airola, Paavo, N.D., Ph.D. *How to Get Well.* Phoenix, AZ: Health Plus Publishers, 1974.

American Orthopaedic Foot and Ankle Society. (For contact information, see under Helpful Organizations on page 180.)

American Podiatric Medical Association. (For contact information, see under Helpful Organizations on page 180.)

Byers, Dwight C. *Better Health with Foot Reflexology.* St. Petersburg, FL: Ingham Publishing, Inc., 1987.

Castleman, Michael. *The Healing Herbs.* Emmaus, PA: Rodale Press, Inc., 1991.

Christopher, John R., Dr. *School of Natural Healing.* Springville, UT: Christopher Publications, Inc., 1976.

Colt, George Howe, and Anne Hollister. "The Magic of Touch." *LIFE Magazine,* August 1997.

Dougans, Inge, with Suzanne Ellis. *The Art of Reflexology.* Rockport, MA: Element Books, Inc., 1992.

Ellis, Joe, D.P.M. "Feet First." *Runner's World,* February 1997.

Garland, Sarah. *The Complete Book of Herbs & Spices.* New York, NY: The Viking Press, 1979.

Garrison, Robert H., Jr., M.A., R.Ph., and Elizabeth Somer, M.A., R.D. *The Nutrition Desk Reference.* New Canaan, CT: Keats Publishing, Inc., 1985.

Gerson, Joel. *Standard Textbook for Professional Estheticians.* Bronx, NY: MILADY Publishing Corporation, 1986.

Green, James. *The Herbal Medicine Maker's Handbook.* Forestville, CA: Wildlife & Green Publications, 1990.

Hampton, Aubrey. *Natural Organic Hair and Skin Care.* Tampa, FL: Organica Press, 1987.

Inkeles, Gordon, and Murray Todris. *The Art of Sensual Massage.* New York, NY: Simon & Schuster, Inc., 1972.

Kirschmann, John D., and Lavon J. Dunne. *Nutrition Almanac.* 2nd ed. New York, NY: McGraw-Hill Book Company, 1984.

Lighthall, J.I. *The Indian Household Medicine Guide.* Memphis, TN: Flying Eagle Enterprises, 1883 & 1996.

Lust, John B., N.D., D.B.M. *The Herb Book.* New York, NY: Bantam Books, 1974.

McVicar, Jekka. *Herbs for the Home.* New York, NY: Penguin Books USA, Inc., 1995.

Meyer, Clarence. *American Folk Medicine.* Glenwood, IL: Meyerbooks, 1973.

Meyer, Clarence. *Herbal Recipes.* Glenwood, IL: Meyerbooks, 1978.

Milady's Art and Science of Nail Technology. Albany, NY: MILADY Publishing Company, 1992.

Norman, Laura. *Feet First: A Guide to Foot Reflexology.* New York, NY: Simon & Schuster, Inc., 1988.

Ody, Penelope. *The Complete Medicinal Herbal.* New York, NY: Dorling Kindersley Limited, 1993.

O'Keefe, Linda. *Shoes: A Celebration of Pumps, Sandals, Slippers & More.* New York, NY: Workman Publishing Company, Inc., 1996.

Page, Linda Rector, N.D., Ph.D. *How to Be Your Own Herbal Pharmacist.* Carmel Valley, CA: Healthy Healing Publications, 1991.

Pedorthic Footwear Association. (For contact information, see under Helpful Organizations on page 180.)

Pritt, Donald S., D.P.M., and Morton Walker, D.P.M. *The Complete Foot Book.* Garden City Park, NY: Avery Publishing Group, 1996.

Rodale's Illustrated Encyclopedia of Herbs. Emmaus, PA: Rodale Press, Inc., 1987.

Schering-Plough HealthCare Products, Inc. (For contact information, see under Helpful Organizations on page 180.)

Taber, Clarence Wilbur. *Taber's Cyclopedic Medical Dictionary, Edition 13.* Philadelphia, PA: F.A. Davis Company, 1977.

Weisenfeld, Murray F., D.P.M., and Barbara Burr. *The Runner's Repair Manual.* New York, NY: St. Martin's Press, 1980.

Weiss, Gaea, and Shandor Weiss. *Growing & Using the Healing Herbs.* Emmaus, PA: Rodale Press, Inc., 1985.

Winter, Ruth. *A Consumer's Dictionary of Cosmetic Ingredients.* New York, NY: Crown Publishers, Inc., 1984.

Worwood, Valerie Ann. *The Complete Book of Essential Oils & Aromatherapy.* San Rafael, CA: New World Library, 1991.

Resources

HERBS & SUPPLIES

The American Botanical Pharmacy
P.O. Box 3027
Santa Monica, CA 90408
Info: (310) 453-1987
Orders: (888) 437-2362
Organically grown and wild harvested herbal preparations and high-quality powdered cayenne pepper. Highly recommended! Free catalog.

Aura Cacia
P.O. Box 299
Norway, IA 52318
(800) 437-3301
Source for superior quality essential oils and related items. Free catalog.

Champlain Valley Apiaries
W.A. Mraz
Box 127
Middlebury, VT 05753-0127
(800) 841-7334
FAX (802) 388-1653
Excellent source for reasonably priced raw honey, maple syrup, and beeswax. Free brochure.

Christopher Publications
P.O. Box 412
Springville, UT 84663
(801) 489-4254
FAX (801) 489-8341
Newsletter and herb books with titles by Dr. John R. Christopher. Free brochure.

Dr. Christopher's Original Formulas
1195 Spring Creek Place
Springville, UT 84663-0777
(801) 489-8787
(800) 453-1406
FAX (801) 489-7207
Herbs, syrups, tinctures, balms, teas, medicinal oils, essential oils, and nutritional supplements. Free brochure.

Dry Creek Herb Farm and Learning Center
13935 Dry Creek Road
Auburn, CA 95602
(530) 878-2441
FAX (530) 878-6772
High-quality organically grown herbs. Free catalog.

FIRM Direct
P.O. Box 5917
Columbia, SC 29250
(800) THE-FIRM
Excellent aerobic weight-training video tapes and exercise equipment. Free catalog.

Flying Eagle Enterprises
3125 S. Mendenhall #422
Memphis, TN 38115-4802
(800) 582-3713
FAX (800) 284-7108
Books about Native American history and herbal usage. Free book list.

The Great Cape Cod Herb, Spice & Tea Co.
Stephan Brown, Owner, Herbalist & Naturopathic Consultant
2628 Main Street
P.O. Box 1206
Brewster, MA 02631
(508) 896-5900
FAX (508) 896-1972
e-mail: ginkgo@greatcape.com
Website: www.greatcape.com
Complete old-fashioned herbal apothecary. Free catalog.

Jean's Greens Herbal Tea Works!!
119 Sulphur Spring Road
Norway, NY 13416
(315) 845-6500
(888) 845-TEAS
FAX (315) 845-6501
e-mail: jean@jeansgreens.com
Website: www.jeansgreens.com
Jean Argus, owner, is a terrific lady. Her new shop carries just about everything you'll need for the recipes in this book, the service is friendly and fast, and the prices are reasonable. Free catalog.

Liberty Natural Products
8120 SE Stark
Portland, OR 97215
(503)256-1227
Offers a variety of herbal extracts, essential oils, and natural products; catalog available.

LorAnn Oils
4518 Aurelius Road
P.O. Box 22009
Lansing, MI 48909-2009
(888) 456-7266
FAX (517) 882-0507
Homemade candy and soap supplies, essential oils, zinc oxide powder, Epsom salts, base oils, wax, fragrance oils, etc. Free catalog.

Meyerbooks
Attn: David Meyer
P.O. Box 427
235 W. Main Street
Glenwood, IL 60425
(708) 757-4950
A wide selection of herb books ranging from new to centuries-old reproductions. Free brochure.

Mountain Rose Herbs

20818 High Street
North San Juan, CA 95960
(800) 879-3337
FAX & info. (916) 292-9138
e-mail: mtrose@asis.com
Website: www.botanical.com/mtrose
*Herbs, herb seeds, oils, essential oils,
bottles, jars, hair/skin care products,
tinctures, salves, teas, and Cap M Quik
capsule filler. Free catalog.*

Original Swiss Aromatics

P.O. Box 6842
San Rafael, CA 94903
(415) 459-3998
FAX (415) 479-0614
*Superior quality "genuine & authentic"
(g&a) and vintage essential oils. They
specialize in providing absolutely genuine essential oils from farmers and dis-
tillers. Their oils are guaranteed pure
and suitable for aromatherapy work or
other healing modalities. Free catalog.*

Pacific Institute of Aromatherapy

P.O. Box 6723
San Rafael, CA 94903
(415) 479-9121
FAX (415) 479-0119
*Superior quality essential oils and in-
depth aromatherapy certification cor-
respondence courses and seminars.
Free catalog.*

Pines International, Inc.

P.O. Box 1107
Lawrence, KS 66044-8107
(800) MY-PINES
FAX (913) 841-1252
Website: www.wheatgrass.com
*Organically grown wheat and barley
grass, select herb powders, and supple-
ments. Free catalog.*

Plant Talk Herbal Products

Andrea Murray, Certified
Herbalist/Reflexologist
38 Foreside Road
Cumberland, ME 04110
(207) 781-3736
*Herbal tinctures, footbath salts, salves,
syrups, and teas.*

September's Sun Herbal Soap Co.

Stephanie Tourles, Owner,
Lic. Aesthetician, Herbalist, Author
P.O. Box 772
W. Hyannisport, MA 02672
(508) 862-9955
FAX (508) 778-9262
*Handmade herbal/grain-based soaps,
herbal body products, and personally
autographed herb books. Send SASE
for free product brochure.*

Simpler's Botanical Co.

Box 39
Forestville, CA 95436
(800) 652-7646
FAX (707) 887-7570
*Aromatherapy–grade essential oils,
tinctures, glycerites, herbal skin care
products, and books. Free catalog.*

Sunburst Bottle Co.

5710 Auburn Blvd. #7
Sacramento, CA 95841
(916) 348-5576
FAX (916) 348-3803
Website: www.planetmall.com/sunburst
*Every type of bottle or jar you'll ever
need. Reasonably priced. Free catalog.*

Super Blue Green™ Algae
Stephanie Tourles, Independent Distributor #457-47-7064
P.O. Box 772
W. Hyannisport, MA 02672
(508) 862-9955
FAX (508) 778-9262
This wild-harvested algae has changed my life and my health for the better! Call or write for further information. To receive information, a SASE is appreciated. Money-back guarantee!

The Vermont Country Store
P.O. Box 3000
Manchester Center, VT 05255-3000
(802) 362-2400
FAX (802) 362-0285
A country store carrying all-cotton hosiery, natural skin/body care products, Dr. Scholl's Exercise Sandals, and many other interesting items. Free catalog.

The Vitamin Shoppe
4700 Westside Avenue
North Bergen, NJ 07047
(800) 223-1216
FAX (800) 852-7153
Vitamins, minerals, herb products, and foot care products. Free catalog.

HELPFUL ORGANIZATIONS

American Academy of Podiatric Sports Medicine (an affiliate of the American Podiatric Medical Association)
1729 Glastonberry Road
Potomac, MD 20854
(800) 438-3355
Call for information on sports-related foot health topics.

American Orthopaedic Foot and Ankle Society
1216 Pine Street, Suite 201
Seattle, WA 98101
A group of orthopaedic surgeons who are specialists in the care of diseases and deformities of the foot and ankle. Send for free information on foot care.

American Podiatric Medical Association
9312 Old Georgetown Road
Bethesda, MD 20814
(800) 366-8227
Call for consumer information literature on a variety of foot health topics.

American Reflexology Certification Board
P.O. Box 620607
Littleton, CO 80162
Contact them for certified reflexologist referrals or for information on how to become certified if you're experienced in reflexology.

Herb Research Foundation
1007 Pearl Street, Suite 200
Boulder, CO 80302
(303) 449-2265
Source for scientific botanical information on herbs. Great magazine! Call for membership information.

International Institute of Reflexology
5650 1st Avenue North
P.O. Box 12642
St. Petersburg, FL 33733
(813) 343-4811
Free training seminar information and certified reflexologist referrals.

National Shoe Retailers Association
9861 Broken Land Parkway, #255
Columbia, MD 21046-1151
(410) 381-8282
(800) 673-8446
Provides a listing of shoe retailers who carry footwear in hard-to-find sizes and widths.

Northeast Herbal Association
P.O. Box 10
Newport, NY 13416
(315) 845-6060
e-mail: neha.jeansgreens.com
Organization dedicated to increasing networking and education opportunities of its members. Write for membership information.

Pedorthic Footwear Association
9861 Broken Land Parkway #255
Columbia, MD 21046-1151
(410) 381-7278
(800) 673-8447
Provides a listing of board certified pedorthists in your area.

Reflexology Center
Andrea Murray, Certified Reflexologist/Herbalist
Scarborough Professional Center
136 Route One
Scarborough, ME 04074
(207) 885-5823
Foot and hand reflexology practitioner and herbalist.

Sage Mountain
P.O. Box 420
E. Barre, VT 05649
(802) 479-9825
Offers an outstanding herbal home study course by renowned herbalist Rosemary Gladstar. I highly recommend it! Free brochure.

Schering-Plough HealthCare Products, Inc.
110 Allen Road
Liberty Corner, NJ 07938-0276
(908) 604-1836
FAX (908) 604-1948
Manufactures Dr. Scholl's foot care products and will send you their foot care brochures upon request.

The School of Natural Healing
P.O. Box 412
Springville, UT 84663
(800) 372-8255
(801) 489-4254
FAX (801) 489-8341
e-mail: snh@qi3.com
Website: www.webnetex.com/snh
Offers a comprehensive herbal correspondence course based on the teachings of renowned herbalist Dr. John R. Christopher.

SHOE SOURCES

Birkenstock
P.O. Box 6140
Novato, CA 94948
(800) 761-1404
Call for free mail-order catalog or for a store near you. Their catalog contains all styles manufactured.

Brown Shoe Co. (manufacturer for Naturalizer Shoes)
8300 Maryland Avenue
P.O. Box 354
St. Louis, MO 63166
Consumer Care Dept.: (800) 766-6465
to find a retailer near you.
FAX (314) 854-2037
Website: www.naturalsport.com (for comfort sport shoe information)
Women's comfort dress, casual, and athletic shoes. Free catalog.

Easy Spirit Division
Nine West Group, Inc.
1 Eastwood Drive
Cincinnati, OH 45227-1197
(800) EASY-242
FAX (513) 527-4003
Women's comfort dress, casual, and athletic shoes. Free catalog.

Gempler's, Inc.
100 Countryside Drive
P.O. Box 270
Belleville, WI 53508
(800) 332-6744
FAX (800) 551-1128
Offers all types of weatherproof boots and socks for men and women. Free catalog.

Lands' End
1 Lands' End Lane
Dodgeville, WI 53595
(800) 356-4444
FAX (800) 332-0103
Website: www.landsend.com
Offers natural fiber socks and limited footwear in addition to their traditionally styled clothing. Their shoes are designed with style, comfort, and the anatomy of the foot in mind. Free catalog.

L.L. Bean
Freeport, ME 04033-0001
(800) 221-4221
FAX (207) 552-3080
Website: www.llbean.com
Carries Birkenstock, Stegmann Bavarian Wool Clogs, boots, and their own brands of comfortable shoes, brand name athletic shoes, and natural fiber socks, plus many other items. Free catalog.

New Balance Athletic Shoe, Inc.
61 N. Beacon Street
Boston, MA 02134
(800) 343-1395
FAX (617) 783-5152
Specializes in men's and women's athletic shoes in a wide range of sizes and widths.

Road Runner Sports
6150 Nancy Ridge Drive
San Diego, CA 92121
(800) 551-5558
FAX (800) 453-5443
Website: www.roadrunnersports.com
Everything for the runner or walker. Free catalog.

WearGuard
141 Longwater Drive
Norwell, MA 02061
(800) 388-3300
FAX (800) 436-3132
Website: www.wearguard.com
Socks and work boots. Free catalog.

Wissota Trader
1313 First Avenue
Chippewa Falls, WI 54729-1499
(800) 833-6421
FAX (715) 723-2169
Many national brands of quality comfort shoes in regular and hard-to-fit sizes. Free catalog.

INDEX